"*The Caregiver's Path* is a book that speaks give readers the tools they need to give the care we all want and deserve. Highly recommended."

—HARRY R. MOODY, PHD, director of academic affairs, AARP

"This is a well-written book, full of practical advice about making difficult life and death decisions. The author has been there as a caregiver and understands well the dilemmas that often need to be faced at times of crisis. Well worth reading cover to cover and/or using it for reference."

—MOIRA FORDYCE, MD, MB CHB, FRCPE, AGSF, geriatrician; adjunct clinical professor, Stanford University School of Medicine Chair; Executive Committee, California Coalition for Caregivers

"The first thing that impressed me about this book is how clearly the fourteen chapters are summarized in the table of contents. Practical questions that readers might be considering are presented with general topics and stories they can anticipate. Caregivers, especially experienced ones like author Viki Kind, appreciate this convenient and informative approach. Readers are also told why the book is needed and how to use it.

Having set a user-friendly tone, the author introduces tools and strategies to empower caregivers, healthcare professionals, patients, and others. She walks readers through the healthcare maze of medical terms, forms, decisions, burnout, joys, death, and grief. Interesting examples of ordinary people bridging gaps between inexperience and practice in their roles as caregivers are given. Captivating stories add layers of useful information readers can use later as they create stories in their own lives. All this is done in the framework of ongoing respect for everyone involved in the caregiving process, especially patients.

Specific ways to positively enhance end-of-life experiences are explained in a manner that adds comforting reassurance to a topic many find difficult. Guidance for Advanced Directives, hospice care, and the dying process, including treatment of the mentally disabled, is shared with a needed candor. Additional resources, an appendix, glossary, and index complete Viki Kind's noteworthy efforts to educate and encourage proactivity among readers facing caregiving and other healthcare challenges.

Are you among the growing millions of people who are caregivers now or will be in the future? Do you want to support others in their caregiving roles? Will you need caregiving for yourself? Should you be addressing your end-of-life plans now while you are still able? If you answered yes to any of these questions, you need this book."

—FRANCES SHANI PARKER, author, *Becoming Dead Right: A Hospice Volunteer in Urban Nursing Homes*

"A practical, easy-to-apply method for making tough caregiving decisions with ethics, heart and peace of mind."

—JACQUELINE MARCELL, author of *Elder Rage* and host of *Coping with Caregiving* radio show

"As an elder law attorney, I get questions from caregivers regarding how to make decisions every day. I thought I knew most of the answers—that is until I read Viki's book, *The Caregiver's Path to Compassionate Decision Making*.

Viki obviously has a tremendous amount of technical knowledge on the issues of decision making for someone who cannot make those decisions. However, what really led me to love this book were the personal and practical stories she tells to fantastically illustrate each and every point. Her technical explanations of the points are excellent, but then the real-life-situation discussions really help you know the issues and understand how they work.

Viki's presentation of the material is also very friendly. She walks the reader through the decision making process step by step with questions that the reader would ask or should be asking. Viki then discusses the issues and answers the questions and shows why they are relevant to all other issues. The questions she presents are questions that I know she has been asked thousands of times and are the same questions I have been asked thousands of times. I learned from her answers, as I am sure you will.

I, as a Certified Elder Law Attorney, learned a tremendous amount from this book. I will have this book on my desk as a reference from now on. I encourage you, as a caregiver or someone who advises caregivers, to get this book and use this book."

—H. TODD WHATLEY, JD, Certified Elder Law Attorney, LLM Elder Law, adjunct professor of law, University of Arkansas School of Law

"Finally an insightful and, most importantly, easy-to-understand guide for caregivers navigating the difficult, yet oftentimes heartwarming landscape of caring for their aging parents. Viki Kind has written a practical 'brass-tacks' guide of what you need to make the best decisions for your elder loved one, and she has done it with the compassion and skill you can trust when making these difficult choices. Bravo!"

—JILL GILBERT, cofounder and former CEO, GilbertGuide.com; coproducer, Digital Health @ CES 2011

"Viki Kind offers useful guidance for families and friends of people who are seriously ill. Drawing on her rich experience, she provides instructive questions, helpful suggestions and sometimes simple relief for people facing some of life's toughest situations."

—STEPHEN KIERNAN, author of *Last Rites: Rescuing the End of Life from the Medical System*

The

Caregiver's Path *to* Compassionate Decision Making

MAKING CHOICES FOR THOSE WHO CAN'T

VIKI KIND, MA

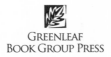

GREENLEAF
BOOK GROUP PRESS

This book is intended as a reference volume only, not as a medical manual. The information given here is designed to help you make informed decisions. It is not intended as a substitute for any treatment that may have been prescribed by a doctor. If you suspect that you or a loved one have a medical problem, you should seek competent medical help. You should not begin a new health regimen without first consulting a medical professional.

Published by Greenleaf Book Group Press
Austin, Texas
www.gbgpress.com

Distributed by Greenleaf Book Group LLC

For ordering information or special discounts for bulk purchases, please contact Greenleaf Book Group LLC at PO Box 91869, Austin, TX 78709, 512.891.6100.

Design and composition by Greenleaf Book Group LLC
Cover design by Greenleaf Book Group LLC

Publisher's Cataloging-In-Publication Data (Prepared by The Donohue Group, Inc.)
Kind, Viki.
    The caregiver's path to compassionate decision making : making choices for those who can't / Viki Kind. -- 1st ed.
    p. ; cm.
    Includes bibliographical references and index.
    ISBN: 978-1-60832-041-7

    1. Caregivers. 2. Care of the sick--Decision making.
    3. Care of the sick--Psychological aspects. 4. Older people--Care. I. Title.
    RT61 .K36 2010
    649.8   2010922760

Part of the Tree Neutral™ program, which offsets the number of trees consumed in the production and printing of this book by taking proactive steps, such as planting trees in direct proportion to the number of trees used: www.treeneutral.com.

Printed in the United States of America on acid-free paper

10 11 12 13 14 15   10 9 8 7 6 5 4 3 2 1

First Edition

TreeNeutral

*Dedicated to all of us who are trying
so hard to do right by our loved ones*

A portion of the proceeds from this book will go to some of the
non-profit organizations that support the groups mentioned in this book.

Contents

The Day My Dad Was Shot in the Dementia Unit
What Should You Do First?
Getting Your Loved One Professionally Evaluated
Determining Capacity
Core Question #1: Does the individual have the ability
to make his or her own decisions? Does he or she have
decisional capacity?
How Long Will This Inability to Think and Communicate
Last?
Core Question #2: If the person is not able to speak for
him- or herself, how long will it last?
Fluctuating Capacity

Learning the Tools

Using the Right Framework to Build a Good Decision
Decision Making Framework
Core Question #3: Was the individual able to speak for
him- or herself in the past?
Autonomy
Substituted Judgment
Using the Platinum Rule
Questions to Use with Substituted Judgment
Making the Decision
Who Should Make the Decisions?
Core Question #4: Who should make the decisions when this
person can't?
When the Person Making the Decisions Is Getting It Wrong

Who Will Decide?
How to Use the Best Interest Standard
Which Patients Will Need the Best Interest Standard?
Who Is the Unbefriended or Unrepresented Patient?
Do You Know Which Framework to Use?

How Old Is Your Loved One Mentally?
Core Question #5: About how old is the person
    developmentally? What is his or her mental age?
The Shared Decision Making Model

The Sliding Scale for Decision Making
The Danger of Using This Tool Incorrectly

How the Assent Tool Works
Should Your Loved One Participate in the Decision Making
    Process, and If So, How Much?
The Assent Tool
Obtaining the Person's Assent or Dissent
The Problem with Assent
Does No Mean No?
Improving Communication When Asking for Assent
Be Careful When You Try This with Your Loved One
Fighting for Control
Babying Your Loved One
When the Person's Developmental Age Is Fourteen to
    Seventeen Years Old

Testing Our New Knowledge
5 Core Questions Flowchart

Using the Tools in Real Life

The End of Life

What Does Your Loved One Deserve?
Making Decisions about CPR and DNR
If I Say, "No CPR," Does That Mean Everything Stops?
When Your Loved One Gets CPR Against Her Will
When Your Loved One Said to Do Everything, but
    Everything Isn't Possible
What Is the Difference Between Palliative Care, Comfort
    Care and Hospice Care?
How Do I Get My Loved One on Hospice?
When the Doctor Won't Put Your Loved One on Hospice
Hospice Information for Doctors
Communicating with the Dying
The Journey Through the Early Days of Dying
The Journey Through the Final Days of Dying
Did I Matter?
Discrimination at the End of Life for the Mentally Disabled

The Day My Mom Died

Introduction

This is the book I wish I had when I was twenty-one and my mom had a massive stroke. I was thrown into a world I knew nothing about—the world of medicine. I felt helpless and all alone although I wasn't actually alone. I had three wonderful brothers, but we were all inexperienced when it came to caring for and making decisions for someone who had become disabled, both physically and mentally. I was worried not only about my mom's health but also about making the right decisions for her.

My mom was an energetic and social person. If you had asked her what she would have wanted after her stroke, she would have said, "I don't want to live like this." But her doctor never asked what my mother would want, and we didn't know we were supposed to speak up for her. So for many years, my mom got what the doctor wanted for her and not what she would have wanted.

Back then, I didn't know what to do to make sure my mom was respected and protected. Now, I know I could have found a doctor who would have listened to and respected her wishes. I could have asked for help from the hospital's bioethics committee. I now know that there are laws that would have protected my mom. I could have gotten her better care when she came back home. There are so many other things I could have done better. By sharing with you what I have learned, I hope to help you along the path toward making better medical and life decisions for those you take care of.

Today, I work as a clinical bioethicist, a medical speaker and a hospice volunteer. As a bioethicist, I help patients, families and healthcare professionals figure out the right thing to do when a loved one is in a medical crisis. My brother says that I came to my life's work because of what I went through with our mom. He is right, even though I didn't make the connection until he said it years later. All I remember from those early days after my mom's stroke is that I felt overwhelmed, fatigued, frustrated, sad and very uncertain. I now recognize all of these symptoms as caregiver burnout and fatigue.

Maybe resources were available back in 1985, but I was unaware of them and I didn't know where to turn. Our access to information has improved substantially with increased research and new resources available through organizations, books and the Internet. But still, every day I work with families and doctors who don't know what to do when it comes to making decisions for individuals who have lost the capacity to think for themselves.

One of the reasons healthcare professionals and families struggle with patients who have had a stroke or have dementia or some other mental limitation is that nobody taught them what I know. As a bioethicist, I have special tools and strategies to help solve these complicated and difficult situations. I am going to share with you these tools and once you have finished reading this book, you will be able to solve these problems yourself. It won't be difficult. The only trick will be to use the right tool in the right situation. But don't worry, I will teach you an easy way to figure out what tools to use when it comes time. Soon you will feel more informed and confident about making the right decisions for your loved one.

It is amazing how different things can be when you have the right tools. In 1998, I became the caregiver and decision maker for my father. After undergoing double bypass surgery and suffering prostate cancer, he started to show signs of dementia. I had to make many difficult decisions, such as taking his car keys away, putting him in a nursing facility and eventually transferring him to a dementia unit. Because I felt more prepared and capable of handling these decisions, my dad got what he needed and I wasn't as stressed.

One area of caregiver stress comes from not knowing what to do. I want to empower you with the knowledge of how to make better decisions for the person in your life who needs your help. I understand that these kinds of decisions are never easy, but I hope that the tools you are about to discover will make it easier for you. Before we begin this journey together, I want to tell you that my heart is with you. I know it's not easy to do what you have to do on a daily basis. I admire your courage to do right by your loved one.

How to Use This Book

This book can be used to help people who are mentally unable to think and communicate for themselves. The person may have suddenly had a stroke, and things changed overnight. Or the patient may be suffering from Alzheimer's or dementia, and every day there is an ongoing decline in mental and physical abilities. Or perhaps your loved one has brain cancer or has had a traumatic brain injury that has taken away his or her ability to communicate. This book is not just for you to use today; you can use it over the person's lifetime. As the individual's condition changes for better or worse, the tools you will find in this book can be used for any situation. This is what makes this book so special. It is here to help you on all of those in-between days when your loved one is still here and, in some ways, already gone.

The tools you are about to discover are the tools I use daily as a bioethicist. Some of these tools come from adult medicine and two come from pediatrics. You may be surprised that the best gift I will give you when it comes to making decisions for people who are vulnerable or who have lost their voices comes from the world of pediatric ethics. There is profound compassion and respect in healthcare when it comes to making decisions for children. And if you think about it, don't you often feel like you and your loved one's roles have been reversed and you are now the parent?

Please do not think that I am calling the adult a child. I am not. It's just that these pediatric tools work to respect and protect those who are ethically vulnerable. I honor, respect and advocate for the vulnerable person, whether he or she is eight months old or eighty years old. The adult who is losing or who has lost the ability to think and communicate needs your help. This individual is still a person of value and should not be minimized. The point of this book is to keep this person involved in his or her own life and decisions in a way that is still safe. My ultimate goal is to give these adults back their power, dignity and voice by teaching *you* to be a great decision making partner for them.

I have designed this book to be a step-by-step process for caregivers to use. It can also be used by healthcare professionals or anyone who is working with those who have mental limitations. As we go along, I will teach you the strategies you will need and how to use them in real-life situations. These strategies are:

- The Decision Making Framework
- The Shared Decision Making Model
- The Sliding Scale for Decision Making
- The Assent Tool

Depending on how your loved one is doing, you may need to use some or all of these strategies when making decisions. To figure out which tools to use and when, I have provided five core questions you will need to answer as you move through the chapters. These questions are:

1. Does the individual have the ability to make his or her own decisions? Does he or she have decisional capacity?

2. If the person is not able to speak for him- or herself, how long will it last?

3. Was the individual able to speak for him- or herself in the past?

4. Who should make the decisions when this person can't?

5. About how old is the person developmentally? What is his or her mental age?

In chapter 7, I've provided a flowchart on pages 80 and 81 that guides you through the decision making process step by step. The flowchart shows you visually how the core questions and the four tools connect to help you make the best decisions possible for the person in your care. The flowchart is also presented in appendix 1.

One thing I know about patients who have mental disabilities is that over time, things can change. A year after my dad started having dementia, he started to show signs of improvement. As his condition changed, the rules I used to make his decisions needed to change accordingly. The same is true for those individuals who continue to spiral downward mentally. When your loved one's situation changes, you will need to reevaluate and then use the different tools that will apply in the new situation.

Now, let's get started!

1

Starting Down the Decision Making Path

The Day My Dad Was Shot in the Dementia Unit

My dad fluctuated from mild to moderate dementia. He lived in an Alzheimer's/dementia unit, but he was quite high functioning. When he became confused, his delusions would frequently return him to World War II. One day my dad called and told me he'd been shot. He didn't sound like he was in pain, so I began to ask questions. "Where were you shot, Dad?"

He replied, "I've been shot in the stomach, but it's probably not too bad because they were bullets from a small-caliber pistol." (Well, I didn't know what size bullets come from a small-caliber pistol, but since he wasn't too concerned, then neither was I.)

"Are the people who shot you still in the building?"

"I think they're in the hallway," he replied in a frightened voice.

I asked him if it would be okay if I got the nurse to check on his wounds. He said it would be okay, but that she should be careful because the gunmen were still out there.

I called the nurse's station and explained the situation. I said that I thought that my dad was okay but perhaps his description of being shot in the stomach meant that he was having stomach problems and couldn't report the symptoms accurately. She said she would call me after she checked on him.

A few minutes later she called back and said that my dad seemed to be fine although he had again mentioned being shot. I asked, "Could you do me a favor and take out the bullets?" There was silence. I explained to her that my dad wouldn't rest comfortably if he thought the bullets were still in him and maybe she could just push on his belly and tell him that the bullets had popped out. She thought it was a great idea, and she put me on hold while she went to remove the bullets. After a few minutes, she let me know that the bullets were out and he was feeling better.

There was nothing funny about this situation at the time, even though the nurse and I laughed about it days later. For my dad, the bullets were very real, and I wanted to protect him and to make him feel safe.

After the nurse left, Dad said he felt much better, but he was scared because the shooters were still in the building. I told him that I would send in the Special Forces to clear the building of the enemy and that they were so good, he wouldn't see or hear them in the hallway.

When I called back later to check on him, he was relaxed and comfortable. He felt better and was able to get a good night's sleep because I had protected him as he had protected me throughout the years.

Each time my dad would come out of his delusional state, which fortunately lasted only for a few hours at a time, he would say to me, "I think I was confused, right?" I would respond, "Yes, you were, but you're okay now." I realized that it is better to comfort someone with dementia rather than to argue with them or make them feel "wrong." This isn't to say that we shouldn't strive to get people more engaged in reality, but when they reach out and tell us they are suffering, we should do our best to support and reassure them.

My dad died years ago and I still miss him every day. I love telling this story because it reminds me to do whatever I can—even small things—to comfort those I care for.

As you can tell, I have had a lot of experience with caregiving. Some days I had to make the medical decisions for my dad, and sometimes I had to figure out how to take out imaginary bullets. Regardless of the situation, I had to be kind and respectful. I had to use my heart *and* my mind. When my dad told me he had been shot, my heart reminded me to be compassionate and my mind told me to get more information. If I had only listened with my heart, I would have empathized with my dad but not taken any action. When I included my mind, I realized that I didn't know if he was truly hurt or just afraid. I had to ask for help from the nurse so I could get more information. Once I had enough information, I could decide what to do next. It takes our hearts and our minds to make compassionate, respectful and ethical decisions for those we care about.

When faced with difficult decisions, we can't just jump to a conclusion. We have to think through the problem and spend time figuring out what would be the best thing to do. This book is designed as a process that will help you think through the different decisions you need to make. As you journey along the decision making path, I will ask you five core questions and then provide you with questions you can ask yourself when making the decisions for your loved one. I will also provide you with questions you can ask the people taking care of your loved one. This will be the most important part of the process—asking enough questions and asking better questions. As we begin, it may seem like a lot to learn, but don't worry, the information is organized in a way that makes it easy to learn.

What Should You Do First?

The first thing you need to do is to make sure your loved one has lost his or her capacity to think. For some of you, it is very clear that your loved one can no longer think or communicate. For those whose loved ones are in the early stages of some diseases, the answer may not be as clear. You, as the caregiver or family member, may need to get the person evaluated to determine if the individual is losing or has lost his or her capacity.

> **Capacity** is the term used to describe your loved one's ability to think clearly, to understand and process information, and to make well-reasoned decisions. A legal professional would ask, "Is this person mentally competent?" Since we are not judges, we will use the word **capacity**, not **competency**.

Kim is at the doctor's office with her husband, Chet, who hasn't been himself lately. As he tries to fill out the forms, Kim notices that Chet needs help answering questions that should be easy for him to answer. Then, in the exam room, Chet doesn't seem to understand when the doctor tells him he needs surgery, even when the doctor repeats the information twice. When the doctor asks if he wants to have the surgery, Chet nods and says, "Yes." It is unlike him to agree to something as major as surgery without asking a bunch of questions. Over the last few months, Kim has noticed that things seem to be slipping for Chet, but she doesn't want to embarrass him by bringing this up with the doctor. This means that unless the doctor notices, Chet will not be evaluated to see why his mental abilities are slipping.

Unfortunately, Chet and Kim's situation is common. Healthcare professionals are busy, and loved ones aren't sure if what they are seeing at home is worth mentioning. Or the patient may be really good at hiding his limitations. I know the doctor treating my dad didn't recognize his dementia at first because my dad was charming and could still communicate well. Since I knew him well, I recognized that what my dad said didn't make sense, but his stories sounded fine to the doctor.

I was also part of the problem. At first, I did not want to believe my dad's mental capacity was changing. I made excuses for the changes I was seeing. When my dad forgot to take his medications, I bought him a daily pillbox to help him remember. But this didn't help because he couldn't remember to use the pillbox. Later, when he began asking me to write checks for him, I thought he was just getting older and needed a little help. It wasn't until he had a series of falls and emergency room visits that I realized he needed me to speak up so he could get the help he needed. Resistance to acknowledging what is happening to a loved one can be powerful. As caregivers, we have to overcome our denial and find the courage to speak up.

If you see something that doesn't seem right, you need to protect your loved one by telling the doctor. Don't wait for the doctor or someone else to bring it up. Until somebody notices and takes action, your loved one will not get the care he or she needs. The sooner you get the person help, the better the chances that something can be done to improve the situation.

Getting Your Loved One Professionally Evaluated

You may already have a sense of where your loved one is mentally, but it is a good idea for you to get the person a professional evaluation. Make a list of all the changes you have noticed, and bring it to the next appointment. Include even the small changes, even if you aren't sure they are important. Make sure the doctor takes you seriously and listens to your concerns. If this doctor doesn't take you seriously, then find a doctor who will.

You may be wondering what kind of doctor should evaluate your loved one. The age of the person you are caring for will help determine the kind of doctor needed. Your loved one's primary care doctor can make the referral to the appropriate doctors available in your community. The doctor will probably send a younger patient to a neurologist and/or a psychiatrist for an evaluation. For a senior patient, the doctor might refer the patient to a neurologist, a geriatric psychiatrist and/or a geriatrician. If you are fortunate enough to have a geriatric specialist in your area, then get a geriatric evaluation done. This evaluation will include the physical and mental condition of the patient as well as the patient's living conditions. If the doctor tells you that the patient has lost capacity, then make sure to have the doctor give you an approximate mental age for your loved one. (You will be learning more about how the mental age affects the decision making process in chapter 4.)

Depending on what part of the country you live in, there may or may not be specialists available in your area. Or perhaps you can't afford the cost of an additional office visit. You do not have to get an evaluation in order to use the tools in this book. But if you can, I highly recommend that you have your loved one's mental capacity evaluated. There may be an easy answer to why the person seems to have changed so much. Perhaps your loved one is having a reaction to her new medicine. Or perhaps she is forgetting to take her new Alzheimer's medication and this is making her appear to be getting worse. The doctor may find something to make her better or to at least slow the progression of the disease.

While at the doctor's office, you may discover that the patient can be brought back to a higher level of capacity. Perhaps she has an infection that is keeping her from being her normal self. Or maybe there is some new illness that needs to be dealt with and once it gets treated, her ability to think will come back. Every effort should be made to bring her back to full capacity and to give her back her voice.

Determining Capacity

The main goal when determining capacity is to see whether the decision being made makes sense logically based on the values, beliefs, culture and religion of the patient. The patient not only needs to understand what is being said, but also must be able to process the information and explain why he is making the decisions he makes. Just being able to repeat information is not enough; the information has to be understood.

A doctor will perform certain tests, such as the Mini-Mental State Examination or the MacArthur Competence Assessment Tool for Treatment, to determine capacity. The doctor will ask certain questions to see if the patient is able to make a rational decision. A rational decision makes sense when it follows a logical course, such as, "I want to live; therefore, I want the treatment" or "I don't want to live; therefore, I don't want the treatment." An irrational decision would be "I want to live, but I don't want the only treatment that can save my life." In the Chet and Kim example, Chet agreed to the surgery but didn't fully understand what was happening, and therefore he was not making a rational decision. For your loved one, you may see inconsistencies between what he says he wants and what you know he values. The decision needs to be consistent with the values of the patient—not the values of the doctor and not the values of the family members.

The following question is the first of the five core questions, along with some of the common questions doctors ask themselves when evaluating a patient. (To see a flowchart of how the five core questions work together, see chapter 7 and appendix 1.)

Core Question #1: Does the individual have the ability to make his or her own decisions? Does he or she have decisional capacity?

Here are the questions you should ask to help you find the answer to this important question:

- Does the patient realize there is a decision that needs to be made?

- Can the patient understand what is being said about the disease and the treatment options?

- Can the patient understand the consequences of each of the different options, including the option to do nothing?

- Can the patient think about what he or she wants to do based on his or her own values/beliefs and how the choices would affect his or her life?

- Can the patient communicate his or her decision to the doctor and explain why he or she has made this decision? (An alternate means of communication might need to be used.)

You may want to stop and ask yourself these questions right now. If you answered "yes" to *all* of these questions, then your loved one probably has the ability to make his or her own decisions. If you answered "no," "sometimes" or "not sure" to any of these questions, then your loved one may have lost capacity.

Healthcare professionals don't always like the decisions that patients make, but patients are entitled to make a "bad" decision that is "right" for them, if they have capacity. This is not just an ethical rule that is followed within healthcare; it is the law. It is the patient's body and life. This can be difficult for others to accept. I would encourage you to remember that you aren't the one whose body will go through surgery or who will have to take a medication that will make you feel sick; it's the patient's body. And because it is the patient's body, we use autonomy to allow that person to make his or her own decisions. With autonomy, a person with the capacity to make the decision gets to choose from the appropriate medical options, even if others do not like what he or she decides. The good news is that when it comes to your body, you too get to make your own decisions.

Although you may not agree with the decision, you should check to make sure that the process makes sense. If it doesn't make sense, then you need to check on the patient's capacity. But you need to be careful not to jump to the conclusion that a "bad" decision means a person has lost capacity. This is an ethical dilemma that still occurs even though healthcare professionals should know better. Sometimes doctors think that as long as a patient agrees with them, then the patient has capacity. Then, the minute the patient disagrees with the doctor, the doctor says the patient has lost his or her mind. This is an ethical mistake. People are allowed to have their own opinions, including the option of disagreeing with their doctors. If you find your loved one in this situation, make sure that the person is really incapacitated and not just in disagreement with the healthcare team.

How Long Will This Inability to Think and Communicate Last?

Now that you have determined that your loved one is losing or has lost capacity, it is time for the second core question.

Core Question #2: If the person is not able to speak for him- or herself, how long will it last?

This question has three typical answers:

1. Permanently—the person will never regain the ability to make his or her own decisions.
2. Temporarily—the person may get better.

3. Fluctuating capacity—sometimes the person has capacity, and sometimes he or she does not.

I have included this question in the core questions for two reasons. First, if you aren't sure about the answer, you can ask the doctor. The doctor may say it's too soon to tell. But if you can get an idea of how long your loved one will be in this state, you can begin to take action to get your loved one what he or she needs.

The second reason is that you may need to come to terms with what the future may hold. You may be making the decisions for a very long time. As painful as this might be to think about, it is important that you don't get caught up in dealing with the day-to-day issues and forget about the long-term needs of your loved one. You may need to make plans not only for how you will be handling the next ten weeks but for how you will handle the next ten years. I am not saying this to worry you. I am hoping that by asking the "how long" question, you will learn where to focus your problem-solving efforts.

Fluctuating Capacity

Fluctuating capacity is when a person has some good days with full capacity to think and then on other days loses this capacity. My dad had vascular dementia, and sometimes he could make his own decisions and sometimes he couldn't. There were also times when he could make some types of decisions but not others. The types of decisions he could make depended on what part of his brain had been affected and how it was affecting his decision making ability that day.

Let me give you another example. A patient has been recovering in the hospital and has been doing well. But for the last day or so she has had terrible pain. The doctor prescribes a pain medication that makes the patient very sleepy. While she is on the pain medication, the patient does not have the ability to communicate her wishes. As she recovers, her ability to make decisions will also recover.

Fluctuating capacity is often seen with some forms of mental illness. Some days the person can be functioning well and be fully capable of handling her life. Then the person can have a number of bad days. The condition of the patient goes back and forth, so her ability to make decisions also flips back and forth. The best way to tell if a person is having a good-capacity day or a bad-capacity day is to see if she can pass the questions in core question #1.

When patients have fluctuating capacity, certain problems can occur in the hospital. When the patient is having a bad mental day, the caregivers or healthcare team may forget to respect what this person voiced on the good days. Or maybe the caregivers or healthcare team are so used to having to make the decisions that they forget to ask the person's opinion on a good day. Either way, the patient doesn't have a voice in the decision making process, and what is important to her is not being respected. This is not okay. You need to make the effort to catch the person on her good days so you can find out what she would want you to decide on the bad days. Then respect those requests on the days when she can't speak for herself. Yes, this might take more time or might be more difficult, but you owe it to your loved one to make sure her voice is heard.

Now that you understand the process of determining capacity, it's time to learn the first part of the decision making process.

LEARNING THE TOOLS

2

The Decision Making Framework

There are four parts to the decision making process. First you will learn how to use the Decision Making Framework as the foundation for building a good decision. Then, you will learn the three tools that you will need for building the rest of your decision. The three tools are the Shared Decision Making Model, the Sliding Scale for Decision Making, and the Assent Tool. Later you will learn how the tools work together to build a good decision.

Using the Right Framework to Build a Good Decision

When building a house, having the right tools and materials ready, and then doing things in the right order, matters. If you try to build a house starting with the roof, it won't work. You have to build a house from the bottom up or it won't hold together. Just like you need a solid foundation to build a house, you need the right framework to start building your good decision. The foundation you will be using is the Decision Making Framework. The Decision Making Framework has three parts you can choose from: Autonomy, Substituted Judgment, and the Best Interest Standard. You will need to choose the correct framework option for the person in your care in order to be respectful of the individual's wishes. This is the starting point for all good decision making.

Figure 2.1: Decision Making Framework

Framework	Ranking	Definition
Autonomy	Best option	Autonomy means a person with decisional capacity is allowed to make decisions about what will happen to his or her own body.
Substituted Judgment	Second-best option	Substituted Judgment is used when the person has lost decisional capacity. Someone else will make the decisions based on the *patient's values and wishes*.
Best Interest Standard	Third-best option	A decision maker and/or the healthcare team, who may or may not know the patient, will make the decision without the benefit of knowing what the patient would want. What would a generic or reasonable person want in this situation?

When we use the Decision Making Framework to make a good ethical decision, we want to choose the best option available. This is why the options have been ranked in order of preference. The best option is Autonomy, the second-best choice is Substituted Judgment and the third, and worst, option is the Best Interest Standard. So which of these frameworks are you going to use? The answer lies in the third core question.

Core Question #3: Was the individual able to speak for him- or herself in the past?

1. Yes, the individual used to be fully capable and was able to express his or her own wishes, but now...

   Scenario A: The person is just starting to lose the ability to make his or her own decisions. Answer: The person may still be able to make his or her own decisions. If the person still has enough capacity, you will use **Autonomy**. When the individual is no longer able to think rationally, then you will use **Substituted Judgment**.

   Scenario B: The person has lost most of the ability to make his or her own decisions. Answer: You are going to use **Substituted Judgment**.

   Scenario C: The person has lost all of the ability to make his or her own decisions. Answer: You are going to use **Substituted Judgment**.

2. No, the person never had full capacity, but he or she has been able to express preferences about some day-to-day things. Answer: You are going to use some **Substituted Judgment** and lots of the **Best Interest Standard**.

3. No, the person was never able to express any opinions or values. Answer: You are going to use the **Best Interest Standard**.

4. I don't know because I don't know anything about this person. Answer: You are going to use the **Best Interest Standard**.

As you begin to learn more about these different frameworks, you will know if you have picked the right framework to use for your loved one. Let's begin with autonomy.

Autonomy

Autonomy only works with people who have the capacity to make their own decisions. If you have determined that your loved one still has capacity, then this is the correct decision making option. Autonomy means that the person who has the capacity to make decisions is able to make her own decisions. The person gets to say what should be done to her body.

When I went to my doctor to talk about my injured back, my doctor told me what options were available to help me get better. He said I could try physical therapy, have a cortisone injection in my back, or just wait and see if it got better over time. Because I had the ability to think for myself and to make my own decisions, I was able to choose what I wanted to do. I definitely wanted to postpone having a needle put into my back, so I told my doctor that I wanted to try physical therapy. I got to think about the different options I was given and then make my own decision.

Here are some of the patients' rights that come with using autonomy:

- Patients have the right to receive all the information they need to make a good decision.
- Patients have the right to make their own decisions.
- Patients have the right to refuse treatments they do not want.
- Patients do *not* have the right to demand treatments that will be medically ineffective or are medically inappropriate for their condition.

It is important to realize that there are limits to a patient's rights. A patient is limited to asking only for treatments that will benefit him. This limitation makes sense. It would be pointless, and potentially harmful, to provide a treatment or medication that would not improve the patient's condition.

Keep in mind that autonomy only works with people who have the capacity to make their own decisions. Since you have probably determined that your loved one does not have decisional capacity, you will have to use Substituted Judgment or, possibly, the Best Interest Standard.

Substituted Judgment

A long time ago, I was a substitute teacher. My job was to follow the plans the teacher had left. I wasn't supposed to change the plans and teach what I thought should be taught that day. In fact, I might have lost my job if I had tried to impose my plan instead of following the teacher's plan. This is exactly how

Substituted Judgment works. You are supposed to step into the patient's life and speak with the patient's voice—not your own voice. You are *not* supposed to bring your own agenda, beliefs, values, culture or religion into the situation. Instead, you are supposed to use the patient's beliefs, values, culture and religion. As the decision maker, you are to imagine what the patient would say if he or she were able to wake up, understand what was going on and be able to make his or her own decisions. Here is a question from someone who had to use Substituted Judgment.

Dear Viki,

The doctor just told me I have difficult decisions to make. She said that I have to decide if it is time to let my mom die. Do I want to take my mom off the ventilator? Would my mom want CPR? How can I begin to make such terrible decisions?

My answer:

I am so sorry that you and your mom are in this situation. I am here to help, and I have a gift for you. It is not your decision. You are just the representative of the patient and are supposed to be speaking as if you were the patient herself. You are supposed to use the values of the patient, not your values. The doctor should have asked, "What would your *mom* be telling us if she were able to speak right now? What would your *mom* say about wanting CPR?" The doctor has burdened you by making it seem like it is your choice, but it shouldn't be your choice. You are the substitute filling in for your mother. Different states call this role different terms:

durable power of attorney for healthcare, agent, proxy or *surrogate decision maker*. But no matter what it is called, the rules are the same. The patient's wishes are supposed to be honored.

As the decision maker, you are supposed to consider all that you know about your mom, what she has told you in the past, what her values are, and what would be important to her. Using this information, do your best to make the decision you think your mom would make. What if you realize that your mom would say, "I don't want to live like this. I would rather die"? Then you have to tell the doctor the truth. I can hear you saying, "But I don't want her to die." Of course you don't. But you have a job to do as the decision maker, and it is up to you to be brave. You need to do the respectful and loving thing and tell the doctor what your mom would say, even if it is not what you would choose for your mom yourself. This is the gift you can give your loved one by speaking for her one more time. Otherwise, you are betraying your mom and disrespecting her beliefs and her life. I am not saying this is easy to do, but it is the right thing to do. On the other hand, if your mom would have said, "Keep fighting and don't give up," then you should tell the doctor this. If this is the case, you will have to advocate for your mom and ask for all appropriate medical treatments to be offered. Here is a secret: If you want the doctor to be on your side, do not say, "Do everything." The words *do everything* have become a problem in healthcare, with people demanding treatments that won't benefit the patient and will only increase the patient's suffering. Instead of saying, "Do everything," what you want to say is "My mom would say, 'I want everything that is medically appropriate to be done.'" When you say, "My mom would say," this lets the doctor know you are thinking about your mom's wishes. The words *everything that is medically appropriate to be done* tell the doctor to do everything that would benefit her and help her get better and to not do those treatments that would only harm her.

Here is another concept that will help you understand Substituted Judgment.

Using the Platinum Rule*

You are probably aware of the Golden Rule, which is found in almost every religion: "Treat people as you would like to be treated" or "Do unto others as you would like to be done unto." Developed by Dr. Tony Alessandra, the Platinum Rule is another way to be respectful. It says, "Treat people as *they* would like to be treated" or "Do unto others as *they* would like to be done unto." The Golden Rule assumes that everyone is the same and would want exactly what you would want. But we aren't all alike, and we can get into trouble when we make that assumption.

For example, if someone you know dies and people wanted to comfort you, would you want people to hug you or would you prefer that they did not touch you? I am a hugger, so if I use the Golden Rule, then I would hug you whether you liked it or not. But if I used the Platinum Rule, I would ask you if you could use a hug and depending on what you tell me, I would respect your answer and hug or not hug you.

The Platinum Rule works really well in the United States because we have such a diverse population. We have different religions, cultures, values and basic preferences. Because respecting other people's medical choices is important, if you told me you wanted to live in a terrible condition that I would never want to live in, I would respect your answer, even though I may not agree with it.

Questions to Use with Substituted Judgment

If you know the patient's preferences, then do what he has asked you to do. If he wrote down his wishes, then you should follow what was written. (If you know nothing or very little about this person, then you will need to use the Best Interest Standard that you will learn in the next chapter.)

If you know the person, but you're not exactly sure what he or she would want, ask yourself the following questions:

- What would the patient say if he or she could talk right now?

- Would the patient want to live like this? If not, what condition would the patient be willing to live with?

- Did the patient say anything to you or others in the past that indicates what he or she might want?

- What would the patient say is important to consider when making this decision?

- What personal, religious or cultural beliefs would be important to the patient in this situation?

- If the patient would say, "I want my family involved in making these decisions," or "I would want to do what my family wants me to do," then you can add the family's opinions to the decision making process. If not, you should focus on what the patient would tell you.

- If I don't know what the patient would say, whom should I ask?

- What do I *not* want to admit to myself or to the doctors about what the patient would say about this situation?

- What am I afraid to say aloud?

- What would I want, and how is that different from what the patient would want?

Making the Decision

Not only do you need to ask yourself what the patient would want, you also need to ask the doctor lots of questions until you have enough information to make an "informed" decision. For a complete set of questions you can use when making medical decisions, see chapter 10, "Making the Medical Decisions." For now, just remember that it is your responsibility to be fully informed before you make any decisions.

Once a decision is made, have the physician specify in writing what has been decided. You will be asked to sign a consent form stating that you understand the risks involved and that you are agreeing to the treatment, surgery or procedure for your loved one. After the treatment begins, check in to see how the patient is reacting to the treatment. Is the patient doing better? Did the treatment help? Is it making your loved one worse? If the patient is not receiving the proposed treatment, how is she doing without it? If the treatment is not going as it should, you can change your mind, withdraw the consent and create a new treatment plan.

This is an ongoing process. You will need to continually reevaluate and adjust the plan as the patient's condition changes. Your job won't be done with one good decision. Your job as the decision maker is an active one, and you will need to continue to stay in communication with the healthcare team. Be careful. Too often, doctors, patients or caregivers get going in one direction and forget to change course when the plan stops working. Be willing to say, "We need to stop and make a new decision."

When I think back to when I was twenty-one and having to take care of my mom, I am still sad that I didn't know what I was supposed to do to respect and honor her. I remember my mother telling me when she was healthy that she would never want to live like my grandmother did after my grandmother's stroke. My grandmother had a terrible stroke and lived for a year in a nursing home before she died. She could barely speak. She rarely recognized us and sometimes called us the dog's name. She was bed bound, with no quality of life. I was twelve or thirteen at the time, and every day my mother and I would visit my grandmother. We would have to take a deep breath and hold our noses to make it down the hallway to her room. The smells of cleaning solution and humans were too much to bear. But every day we would visit and every day it was the same. My grandmother was there but already gone.

When my mom had her own stroke, she was paralyzed on one side, but at least she could still talk. She hated being stuck in bed and having to depend on others. She became depressed and gave up trying to get better. We didn't realize it at the time, but my mom also had an undiagnosed mental illness. The combination of the stroke and her mental illness made it difficult for her to make her own decisions. Sure, she could talk and complain, but she wasn't able to look out for herself anymore. Back then, I didn't realize that I needed to protect her and that I was now in charge.

If the doctor had asked me, I would have told her that my mom wouldn't want to live in that condition. She had said over and over again that she wouldn't want to end up like her own mother. But here she was, in almost the exact same situation, without any hope of escaping her body. I didn't speak up or advocate for her, because I didn't know how. If I had known then what I know now, I would have had the courage to do the right thing. I wish I could make it up to her.

It is a truly heroic act to be the decision maker, especially in difficult life-or-death moments. I honor and respect the courage it takes to make these difficult decisions. I know that when it comes time, my own decision maker will have the courage to make the hard choices, even if he doesn't agree with my wishes, because he respects and loves me. It is said that doing the right thing is sometimes the hardest thing. I know you have the courage to step up and become a great decision maker for your loved one.

Who Should Make the Decisions?

At one time or another in your life, you, the caregiver, may need to have someone else make your decisions for you. If you have capacity and can still think and communicate for yourself, then you can write down whom you want to make your decisions for you on a form called an Advance Directive for Healthcare; this is also called a Durable Power of Attorney for Healthcare or a Living Will. (I will use the term Advance Directive for the rest of the discussion.)

The Advance Directive for Healthcare is a form that a person can complete while he or she still has the capacity to think and communicate. This is a written document that indicates what types of medical treatments you would want and whom the doctor should speak to when you are unable to speak for yourself. See appendix 2 for more information about the Advance Directive.

It's okay if you want more than one person to share in the decision making process for you. If your culture says that your family or a group of people should make your decisions, then you will need to write this down ahead of time or else the doctor will ask just one person to make the decisions for you. Or perhaps in your culture, the family should make the decisions for the patient, even when the person still has capacity. If so, the patient will have to let the doctor know that he wants to give his decision making power to someone else. In the United States, the patient with capacity has to give away his decision making power; the family cannot just take it.

Conflicts can arise if the doctor doesn't know whom to talk to. Your family may fight over who should be speaking for you or argue about what they think you would want to have done.

Many times I have seen a family break apart because of disagreements about who should be the decision maker. While the family is battling it out, the patient is vulnerable because nobody is speaking for him. When conflict comes into the hospital room, the patient loses.

Core Question #4: Who should make the decisions when this person can't?

The answer to this question could be any one of the following:

Person specified on the Advance Directive

Conservator or guardian

Spouse

Significant other/partner

Adult child of patient

Parent

Adult sibling

Relative

Friend

Family

Healthcare team

Administrator of the nursing home (in some states)

While this is a general list, the answer really depends on where you live, what the patient has specified and if the court has gotten involved. Each state calls the decision maker by a different name: *surrogate decision maker, agent, proxy* or *durable power of attorney for healthcare.* The laws that determine who should make the decisions also change state by state. For example, the administrator of a nursing home may be allowed to make the decisions in one state, but can't in a different state.

Another rule that varies is the law that dictates a specific hierarchy of decision makers. A hierarchy means there is a legal order to who will be allowed to make the decisions for someone who has lost capacity. You may need to ask the social worker, the bioethics committee or the legal department at the hospital to help you figure out the appropriate laws in your state.

Here is what one hierarchy of decision makers looks like in Florida as of 2010.

1. The judicially appointed guardian of the patient;

2. The patient's spouse;

3. An adult child or a majority of the adult children of the patient who are reasonably available for consultation;

4. A parent of the patient;

5. The adult sibling of the patient or, if the patient has more than one sibling, a majority of the adult siblings who are reasonably available for consultation;

6. An adult relative of the patient who has exhibited special care and concern for the patient and who has maintained regular contact with the patient and who is familiar with the patient's activities, health, and religious or moral beliefs;

7. A close friend of the patient;

8. A licensed clinical social worker who is a graduate of a court-approved guardianship program. Such a proxy must be selected by the provider's bioethics committee and must not be employed by the provider.

So in Florida, if you are the spouse of the patient, you are automatically the decision maker unless the person wrote an Advance Directive stating that he or she wanted someone else to make the decisions. The only other time the spouse wouldn't be the decision maker in Florida is when the court has stepped in and assigned a conservator or a guardian to make the medical decisions for the patient.

In California, the law does not establish a hierarchy of decision makers. What does this mean? Anybody who knows the patient can be the decision maker. It can be the patient's spouse, partner, parent, sibling or friend or anyone else in the patient's life, but there is no specific order as to whom should be chosen. In California, we are told to use the person who knows the patient best and will respect the patient's values and beliefs. This lack of a hierarchy allows flexibility in choosing different people to be the decision maker, but it can also create confusion and conflicts when multiple people think that they should be in charge. For this reason, I strongly encourage anyone who lives in a hierarchy-free state like California to fill out an Advance Directive. (See appendix 2.)

If you are named as the decision maker, you don't have to take on that responsibility. Perhaps you live too far away and can't visit the patient. Or perhaps you know that you won't be able to respect the patient's wishes. You are allowed to say no and the power will move on to a different person. Then you may want to give this book to that person so he or she can learn how to make these important decisions.

When the Person Making the Decisions Is Getting It Wrong

What if you are not the assigned decision maker and you think the person who is making the decisions is getting it wrong? What can you do? Let me start by telling you some gentle ways you can try to help and end by telling you about more assertive ways you can get involved. I encourage you to try the gentle approach first, because the decision maker has control over the patient's healthcare decisions and can limit your ability to visit your loved one.

You can begin by sharing the lessons you learned from this book with the decision maker. The most important piece of information that I share with the families I work with in the hospital is how to use Substituted Judgment in order to respect the values and wishes of the patient.

You should also try to consider the situation from the decision maker's perspective. Perhaps she is exhausted, overwhelmed, in terrible grief or unable to understand all of the complex medical information. All of these can limit someone's ability to think clearly and to make the right decisions. Maybe you can take over some of the caregiving responsibilities so she can get a break. Or maybe you can show appreciation and say, "Thanks, I know this is a lot of work for you." Or perhaps you can give her permission to cry and to grieve. Many people find comfort in caregiver support groups, whether online or in person. (If the decision maker is suffering, it will be more difficult for this person to make good decisions.)

Whatever you do, you should try to partner with the designated decision maker rather than fight with her. Ask, "How can you and I solve this problem together?" Then you and she can begin to solve the problem as a team. Offer to do some research about the medical treatment the doctor is recommending. Be helpful, and she may begin to appreciate your advice.

If the gentle approach doesn't work, then you will need to ask for outside help. At the hospital, the social worker is the first person you should reach out to. This person knows how the medical system works and knows whom you should contact. Another person to ask for help is the nursing supervisor. You can also contact whomever is on call for the bioethics committee or ethics committee. Just call the hospital operator and ask to speak with the bioethics committee. The committee can help whether the issues are within the family or the disagreement is with the healthcare team. Long-term care facilities have ombudsman services and ethics committees to help families resolve difficulties.

When you feel you need to get even more aggressive, you can take the person who is making bad decisions to court and try to get the individual removed from being in charge. The court may assign someone else in the family to take over or may assign a conservator or guardian to take charge. Or the court may do nothing. The court will not remove the person just because you don't like him or you think he is making bad decisions. It will have to be proven that the person is either harming your loved one or going against the expressed wishes of the patient.

These same approaches work when you think the doctor is not doing the right thing. Try to collaborate at first. If that doesn't work, call the ethics committee. If none of these options work, then you can take the doctor or hospital to court. But

really, the best thing to do if the doctor is doing the wrong thing is to fire the doctor. I should have done this with my mom's doctor when she wouldn't respect my mother's wishes. But at the time, I didn't realize that was an option.

How do you fire a doctor? All you have to do is to say that you no longer want the doctor to take care of your loved one. But before you fire the doctor, make sure that you can find someone else who is willing to be your loved one's doctor. If you or the patient is "a problem," you may not find anyone else willing to take on the care of the patient.

3

The Best Interest Standard

It's time to discuss our third framework option, the Best Interest Standard. We use the Best Interest Standard when we don't know what a patient would want or we can't find someone to speak for the person. The Best Interest Standard is most often used by healthcare professionals, especially for those individuals without capacity who have been abandoned by their loved ones and are living in a nursing home. If you are not a healthcare professional, you may need to know how to use the Best Interest Standard if you don't know your loved one well or you can't figure out what he or she would want.

The Best Interest Standard states that the decision maker and/or the healthcare provider, who may or may not know the patient, will make the decision without the benefit of knowing what the patient would want. This is the worst option to use because no one knows the patient's wishes and someone

> One of the saddest things I see in my work is the growing number of people who have been placed in long-term care facilities and have been abandoned by their families and friends. There is terrible neglect when nobody visits, nobody calls and nobody takes the time to make sure good decisions are being made. It breaks my heart that there is no one to speak for them and to protect them.

must guess what is in the best interest of the patient. To do this, the following question must be asked: "What would a reasonable person want in this situation?" or "What would a generic person want?" This is why this standard is the worst option to use. Who is generic? How do we know what a generic person would want?

Who Will Decide?

For healthcare professionals and bioethicists like myself, the Best Interest Standard gives us the most trouble. It is difficult to know if we are making the right decisions when we know so little about a patient. Another problem I see is that many healthcare professionals have not been trained in how to use the Best Interest Standard. Ideally, it is recommended that these types of decisions should be made as a group in order to have a variety of people express their opinions about what a reasonable person would want. It is also best if someone who knows even a little bit about the patient is involved in the process.

Three groups may be involved in making the decisions using the Best Interest Standard.

1. If there are family and friends involved, they will do the best they can to make the decision without having enough information about what the patient would

want. They may be able to use a little Substituted Judgment with the Best Interest Standard, if the patient ever expressed any preferences. If not, they will do the best they can and only use the Best Interest Standard.

2. In some cases, the court will assign a public or private conservator or guardian to protect the patient. This court-appointed person will make the medical and/or financial decisions for the patient. But of course, the conservator probably doesn't know anything about the patient, so the decisions will be based on what a generic person might want. This is a stranger making decisions for another stranger. There is nothing personal or meaningful in this process.

> If you are a conservator or a guardian, I strongly encourage you to visit the patient in person. Oftentimes, the patient's condition has changed dramatically from the last time you saw the individual, and seeing the patient in person will give you valuable information about what should be done.

3. If there isn't a conservator or guardian available, a group of people at the hospital will make the medical decisions for the patient. Sometimes we call this an advocacy team or a moral community. This group usually consists of a doctor, a nurse, a social worker, a chaplain, members of the ethics committee and a community member. As a group, they will make the decisions.

How to Use the Best Interest Standard

If you do know a little bit about the patient, you will want to consider this person's basic preferences. What has he or she liked or disliked in the past? I know these basic preferences won't give you the total answer, but a person with diminished capacity should be allowed to contribute to the decision in any way possible. Ask the person who has been taking care of the patient to help you understand how to best communicate with the individual and if any personal preferences have been expressed. If someone can't speak with words, it doesn't mean that the person can't communicate in other ways. The individual with diminished capacity can still have a voice in his or her life even if unable to make the final decision. (You will learn how to help your loved one do this in the next chapter.)

The following are the steps for using the Best Interest Standard:

1. Ask all the necessary medical questions in order to make an informed decision. (For a complete set of questions you can use when making medical decisions, refer to chapter 10, "Making the Medical Decisions.")

2. Ask quality-of-life questions to determine how the patient's quality of life has changed because of the current medical situation. Will the treatment being considered improve the person's quality of life? Is the patient suffering? What will the decision mean to the patient's future living situation? (An extended discussion of the quality-of-life issues can be found in chapter 12, "Quality of Life and Personal Values.")

3. Once a decision is made, have the physician document the decision. You can always modify the treatment plan or create a new treatment plan based on new information you may receive over time.

4. After making the decision, continually reevaluate and adjust the plan depending on the patient's condition. Stay in communication with the healthcare team. Be careful. Too often, doctors, patients or caregivers get going in one direction and forget to change course when the plan stops working. Be willing to say, "We need to stop and make a new decision." Remember, this is an ongoing process.

Which Patients Will Need the Best Interest Standard?

The Best Interest Standard is used for two groups of people. The first group includes individuals who have never been able to express their values or wishes, such as a child who was born severely mentally disabled or someone who suffered a terrible brain injury at a very young mental age. These individuals' mental abilities never progressed beyond a very young age. The person may be able to express some basic likes or dislikes, such as what he wants to eat or whether he is in pain, but he will not be able to express opinions about important issues. This person can be any physical age, but developmentally, his mental age never progressed to a point at which he would be able to provide us with important information about his preferences.

The second group includes individuals who have been found unconscious or those who have been living in a care facility, and the healthcare team can't find any friends or family members who know them. Or perhaps the family has been found but they have been out of contact with the patient for many years and don't really know this person or are unwilling to make the decisions. Sometimes we call this patient the *unbefriended person* or the *unrepresented person*.

Who Is the Unbefriended or Unrepresented Patient?

The term *unbefriended* or *unrepresented* describes a patient who has no friends or loved ones the doctor can talk to when the patient has lost capacity. Let me tell you what happened to one unrepresented patient.

A seventy-eight-year-old man collapsed at the market and was brought to the emergency room. The social worker assigned to the case looked through the patient's wallet to find out who he was but found only an insurance card and address. The social worker went to the patient's house, talked to his neighbors and made calls to find anyone who might know this individual. But she didn't find anybody.

Because there weren't enough public guardians in this community, the hospital staff scheduled an advocacy team meeting. At the meeting, the social worker shared with us that she hadn't been able to speak to anyone who knew this person. We asked the doctor about the patient's medical condition and were told he was going to die very soon. As we discussed what would be in the patient's best interest, we thought about how we could improve his quality of life and, in this case, the quality of his final days. Our team unanimously agreed that he should be made comfortable, kept out of pain and be allowed to die a peaceful death.

These are really difficult decisions and not the kind that should be made by strangers. But committees or conservators across the nation are making decisions about people they have never met and know very little about. This is not how it's supposed to be. People shouldn't be dying completely alone, silenced by their diseases.

Instead, I hope families reach out and reconnect with those that have been left behind. I realize that sometimes people have fallen out of our lives for a good reason, so I am not saying you should reconnect in every situation. If you don't want to reconnect emotionally with this individual, perhaps you can at least explain to the doctor what this person used to be like before losing capacity. Many times the social worker finds family members who don't want to be the "final" decision maker, but they can offer information and insights that can help the guardian, conservator or advocacy team make better decisions. If you are up to doing a little bit more, then try to visit the patient occasionally.

> Would you want a stranger to be making life-or-death decisions for you? If the answer is "no," then please tell your doctor who he should talk to if you are injured. Then write down the person's name and phone number in your wallet and remember to fill out your Advance Directive (see appendix 2). I don't want you to ever be the unbefriended patient.

If this issue troubles you as it does me, then you may want to consider volunteering at your local long-term care facility or for your hospital's bioethics committee. You could use your voice to protect and respect others as you do with your loved one. The difference a volunteer's visit makes in the life of a nursing home resident is substantial. Just an hour a week can bring joy and comfort to those who have been left behind. And you may discover the joy in connecting with a person who needs you.

Do You Know Which Framework to Use?

Now that you are familiar with the three parts of the Decision Making Framework, you should know which framework to use to begin the decision making process. Now it is time for you to get the tools you will need to build a good decision.

4

The Shared
Decision Making Model

This is the chapter you have been waiting for; this is the first of the two pediatric tools I was telling you about. Of the three tools you will need to learn—the Shared Decision Making Model, the Sliding Scale for Decision Making and the Assent Tool—the first is my favorite. So you can understand why the Shared Decision Making Model tool is so important, let me begin by telling you a story.

Most of the doctors came to my lecture for help with dealing with their patients who have conservators, but one doctor came for help with making decisions for his thirty-year-old mentally disabled sister. After the lecture, he approached me in the hallway and told me how grateful he was—that he understood why things had been going so wrong and why he had been so frustrated when making decisions for her.

He explained that his sister had the mental capacity of an eleven-year-old and that he had been using the decision making tool that works for a person with the mental age of a sixteen-year-old. She had been getting a bigger voice in her decisions than was appropriate for her mental age. He had been using the wrong tool. It was like trying to hammer a nail in with a screwdriver. It just doesn't work. The look of relief on his face was something I will never forget. I would like to share with you what I taught him.

How Old Is Your Loved One Mentally?

If the doctor says your loved one has lost capacity, your next question should be "How old is my loved one developmentally?" or "What is the person's mental age?" *Mental age* refers to the age level at which a person thinks. For example, though a man may be sixty-five years old in age, he may think like a sixteen-year-old or a ten-year-old or a two-year-old. Knowing the person's developmental age is the key ingredient to making good decisions.

Let me show you a different way to think about it. If you are a parent, would you allow your young child to stay home alone? You wouldn't leave a six-year-old home alone; it wouldn't be safe and it's against the law. You might feel comfortable leaving your twelve-year-old home alone and you would almost certainly let your teenager stay home alone. Of course, your decision would depend on the mental maturity of the child, not just his or her physical age.

It works the same way for someone who has lost or is losing capacity. When you picture your loved one, is it safe for this person to stay home alone? Would you leave your loved one in charge of small children who need watching? The answer will depend on the developmental age of your loved one. So here is your last core question.

Core Question #5: About how old is the person developmentally? What is his or her mental age?

Whether you estimated your loved one's mental age or the doctor has given you an approximate age, your answer will fit into one of these categories. These age ranges will help guide you as you begin to use the Shared Decision Making Model.

Zero to six years old

Seven to thirteen years old

Fourteen to seventeen years old

The Shared Decision Making Model tool is used to determine how much your loved one should participate and how big of a voice he or she should have in important life and health decisions. With this tool, you will be able to adjust this process to fit your loved one's mental abilities as they change over time. For those whose loved one has fluctuating capacity, you will need to adjust the age range as your loved one's condition changes each day.

Figure 4.1: The Shared Decision Making Model
How much should my loved one participate in the decision making process?

Approximate Developmental Age	Decision Making Tool	With children, who participates?	With adults, who participates?
Age 0–6	Parental or Decision Maker's Consent or Permission	Parents and the healthcare team should work together to make medical decisions.	The patient's decision maker uses Substituted Judgment or the Best Interest Standard, then makes the decision.
Age 7–13	Assent	Parents, the healthcare team *and* the patient should work together to make decisions, including getting assent from the child (asking for the child's permission, not consent).	The decision maker, with the help of the doctor if needed, talks to the patient about the medical decisions and gets the patient's assent or permission. The decision maker gives the final consent.
Age 14–17	Consent	The patient may have capacity similar to an adult and, if so, the patient's consent should be obtained.	If the patient has enough capacity, the patient uses autonomy and makes the decisions. If not, you move back up one level and use Assent.

Here are the basic guidelines of the Shared Decision Making Model. If the person in your care is in the zero-to-six-year-old age range, you will need to make the decisions for him or her because it wouldn't be safe for the individual to participate in important decisions. If the person is in the seven-to-thirteen-year-old age range, he or she will be able to have a voice in most decisions but will not make the final decision. If the person is in the fourteen-to-seventeen-year-old age range, the individual may have enough capacity to make his or her own decisions. If not, you will want to use the seven-to-thirteen-year-old guidelines.

The ages on the chart are a guideline, not a rule. You can adjust the ages up or down a little bit, but be careful about moving the developmental age too far out of the decision making guidelines that are shown here: You might end up using the tool in the wrong way.

Think about the doctor who had a thirty-year-old sister with the developmental age of eleven. Should his sister be allowed to drive? Perhaps an eleven-year-old would be allowed to drive on a farm because there would be plenty of space and fewer dangers. But an eleven-year-old child in Boston would probably not be developmentally ready to handle the traffic and the dangers. The same goes for making dangerous medical decisions. The more dangerous the decision, the more mental ability the person needs to have.

Earlier, I said that for a while, my dad's dementia became very severe. At that time, he was probably developmentally around age five. He could talk to me and he knew who I was, but he couldn't connect the dots. He couldn't keep track of information long enough to make sense out of things. It wasn't safe for him to make his own important decisions. He could choose what to have for lunch, but it wouldn't have been safe for him to decide if he needed surgery. So while he was the mental age of five, I had to protect him and use the right tools to make his decisions. Later on, his capacity improved and he fluctuated between ages twelve to seventeen developmentally. As he changed, I had to change what tool I used when making decisions. I was grateful to have the Shared Decision Making Model to rely on, because it let me know when to include him in decisions and when to make decisions for him. I was able to keep him safe when he wasn't able to keep himself safe. Knowing how to approach the situation made a difficult situation much easier for me.

Now, let's move on and learn about the next tool, the Sliding Scale for Decision Making, and how it will help us in different situations.

5

The Sliding Scale for Decision Making

The second tool you will be using is the Sliding Scale for Decision Making. This tool tells us that the more serious the risks involved in the decision, the more the person needs the ability to think. For a person with very minimal capacity, she might be able to make decisions about what to wear or what to watch on TV, but it would be dangerous to let her make important medical decisions. The way I remember this tool is that a less risky decision requires less capacity while a more risky decision requires more capacity.

Figure 5.1: The Sliding Scale for Decision Making
The more risky the decision, the more capacity the individual has to have in order to participate in the decision making process

No capacity	A little bit of capacity	Some capacity	Almost full capacity	Full capacity
No decision making	Some small decisions	Daily decisions and some voice in medical decisions, but not life-or-death decisions	Larger voice in important decisions	Full voice in his or her own decisions, including life-or-death decisions

This new tool works together with the Shared Decision Making Model to make sure that we think about (1) the developmental age of our loved one and (2) the risk or danger involved in the decision. And just like remembering to use the right tools to build a house, you will need to use both of these tools together to make the right decision, as in the following example.

Samara's uncle has cancer that has spread to his brain. It was just last week that her uncle was enjoying sitting outside on the porch but now he sleeps almost all the time. Samara is in a state of shock because his condition changed so quickly. He has an approximate mental age of a four-year-old. Samara is the only person around to take care of him, but she thinks she will need to hire a caregiver because she can't keep missing work. At her uncle's last doctor's appointment, the doctor said that he could try one more round of chemotherapy with her uncle.

Should her uncle have a voice in the chemotherapy decision? No. Because her uncle has a mental age of four, it isn't safe for him to make the decision about whether or not he should have more chemotherapy. This decision also comes with lots of risks and side effects. Samara will have to make this decision. Even if her uncle had a slightly higher mental age, it might not be safe for him to make the decisions, considering the risks involved.

This is why we have the Sliding Scale for Decision Making. It helps us figure out which decisions are safe for our loved ones to have a voice in and which ones are not.

The Danger of Using This Tool Incorrectly

When I talk about allowing patients to have a voice based on their mental age, I try to emphasize how important it is to use this tool correctly. If you overestimate or underestimate the individual's capacity, this tool won't work correctly. For example, if you are the kind of parent who lets your very young children make their own decisions and decide what they will do and when, you may be giving them too much power. You may be putting them in danger because they are not able to make rational decisions.

This is incredibly important. If the person doesn't have enough mental capacity to participate, then the person shouldn't be part of the decision making team. It wouldn't be safe. I know this can be difficult to accept because wishful thinking gets in the way. We wish that our loved ones were the way they used to be. Just because we would like them to participate or wish they could, doesn't mean that they should. We have to be realistic about the situation.

When I was taking care of my mom, I was very young and I was uncomfortable taking on the decision making role. Even though I didn't want to be in charge, I had to protect her and make the best decisions I could. I made the same mistakes taking care of my mom that you might be making. I tried to let her make her own decisions, but when she made a dangerous decision, I had to step in and tell her she couldn't have her way. (You can imagine how well that went.) I got into terrible arguments with her because I kept hoping she would magically be able to think again, and I got frustrated when she couldn't. This wishful thinking ended up making it much worse for both of us, and it harmed our relationship.

If I could go back in time, I would begin by figuring out which tools I should have used when helping my mom. I would approach the situation as follows:

1. Using the Decision Making Framework, I would begin down the right path to make my mom's decisions. Because I knew what my mom's wishes were, I would choose Substituted Judgment.

2. Using the Shared Decision Making Model, I would figure out my mom's mental age. I would then determine if she should participate in the decision making process. Looking back, I think I would have put her in the seven-to-thirteen-year-old developmental age range, so she would have been able to have a voice in the decisions that were safe for her to make.

3. Using the Sliding Scale for Decision Making, I would evaluate how risky each specific decision was so I could determine whether my mom should have a voice in the specific decision. For the less dangerous decisions, my mom would have a larger voice, and for the high-risk decisions, I would have made the decisions for her.

So if my mom were going to have a voice in the decision making process, I would have then needed to know how to use our third tool, the Assent Tool. In the next chapter I will explain how to use this final tool.

6

The Assent Tool

You have made it to the last tool you will need to learn, the Assent Tool. Because this is an action tool that you will be using when interacting with your loved one, I want to make sure you get it right. The Assent Tool is used after you have decided that the person is mentally old enough to participate and that it is safe for him or her to have a voice. The Assent Tool will tell you *how* to give the person a voice in the decision making process.

Imagine that your forty-eight-year-old son has the mental capacity of a ten-year-old. He definitely has opinions and is able to express them, but he does not have enough reasoning ability or common sense to make a good decision by himself. Your son wants to move to a new group home because he doesn't like the people where he is living. You are not thrilled about having to go to the effort to find him a new place and to help him move, but you do want him to be happy where he is

> Doctors in adult medicine don't use this pediatric tool very often. In adult medicine, if the individual doesn't have full and complete capacity, then the person is not allowed to make his or her own decisions. If your loved one has less than full capacity, then the doctor will have you, the decision maker, make the decisions and sign the necessary consent forms. Even though the doctor probably won't ask for your loved one's assent, that doesn't mean that you can't personally use this tool to keep the person included the best you can.

living. Should your son have a voice in the decision? Is it safe for him to make this decision? Does he get to make the final decision?

Because this is not a risky or dangerous decision for him to be involved in making and he has a developmental age of ten, he should be able to have a voice in this decision. But he won't get to make the final decision, because you still need to protect him and make sure that the new place will meet his needs and that he will be safe there.

How the Assent Tool Works

The Assent Tool is the other tool that comes from pediatric ethics. The child who has some capacity should be a participant in the decision making process. It would be much easier for pediatricians to just make the decisions with the parent and leave the child out. But there is a deep respect for the child, even though he or she is young, which says that the child should have a small voice in his or her life. This voice grows as the child's ability to think grows. This is exactly what I want you to do for your loved one: Give your loved one an appropriate voice in his or her life, but only to the extent that it makes sense and is safe.

When you ask the person for assent or dissent, a yes or a no, you are asking if he or she agrees with the plan. As you ask for the person's agreement, you will be putting into action the first tool, the Shared Decision Making Model. This is when you share the decision making with your loved one but you aren't giving the person total control. You will also be using the second tool, the Sliding Scale for Decision Making, which reminds us that the more serious the decision, the more capacity the person has to have to be involved. If it is safe for the individual to have a voice in the decision, you will then use the Assent Tool to give the person his or her voice. The Assent Tool works well with those in the seven-to-thirteen-year-old developmental age range.

Should Your Loved One Participate in the Decision Making Process, and If So, How Much?

Here are two examples of the three tools working together for both a non-life-threatening decision and a life-or-death decision.

Figure 6.1: The Assent Tool
A Non-life-threatening Decision

Age 0–6		Age 7–13		Age 14–17
No capacity	A little bit of capacity	Some capacity	Almost full capacity	Full capacity
No participation	No participation	Will ask for the patient's assent or dissent	Will ask for the patient's assent or dissent	Patient can make his or her own decisions.

Figure 6.2: The Assent Tool
A Life-or-Death Decision

Age 0–6		Age 7–13		Age 14–17
No capacity	A little bit of capacity	Some capacity	Almost full capacity	Full capacity
No participation	No participation	Patient will not be allowed to make life-or-death decisions. Will *not* ask for assent, as this is life or death.	Patient can probably make less risky decisions, but will not ask for assent, as this is life or death.	Patient can make life-or-death decisions.

A life-or-death situation doesn't mean that all treatments are worth the chance. Some treatments are risky and have little chance of success, while other treatments may be equally risky but have a greater chance of success. And some treatments may have no chance of working, or the suffering will be so severe from the treatment that it isn't worth it. When decisions are made for children, the treatment has to have a great enough chance of success to justify putting the child through the toxic side effects. Make sure the benefits are worth the risks for your loved one. (For more information, see pages 116–119.)

Obtaining the Person's Assent or Dissent

Here is how assent works. When you ask for the patient's assent, you are asking for permission. The individual is informed about what will happen in terms the person can understand, i.e., what the test, treatment or surgery will feel like and why it is needed. Then, the patient is given a voice or a vote in the decision. The patient can assent (say yes) or dissent (say no). But remember that this is only one vote, not the final vote. The individual is not the final decision maker because he or she doesn't have quite enough capacity to give a full, informed consent.

You, as the decision maker, will have to give the final consent or refusal because you are able to make a rational and well-thought-out decision. (Some people may say that a thirteen-year-old is too old to be included in this range and should be included in the fourteen-to-seventeen-year-old category. For some thirteen-year-olds I would agree, but for others I think assent still applies.) Remember that the Shared Decision Making Model provides a guideline, not an absolute rule. You have to evaluate your loved one's mental ability that day and use whatever category makes sense. Over time, you will be able to tell if the tool is working as you begin to see how it changes your interactions with your loved one. If it isn't working, don't be afraid to try another category. You can keep adjusting which category you use as you deal with the changing mental ability or inability of your loved one.

> The nice thing about using assent is that it reminds us to include the individual. This helps us keep the person from becoming a "third-party patient," where the doctor and the decision maker talk together and forget that the patient is in the room. Do not do this. Instead, remember that even someone with very little capacity should be included as much as possible.

Here are the steps for getting your loved one's assent:

1. Evaluate your loved one's mental age, maturity level, psychological condition and ability to give assent/dissent.

2. If necessary, allow enough time to use an alternate method of communication. You may need to slow down and repeat yourself a number of times. You and your loved one may need multiple meetings with the doctor before the patient can understand what is being discussed. Don't get frustrated, as your loved one is doing the best he or she can to understand.

3. Using developmentally appropriate language (language the patient can understand), give the patient the necessary information about his or her illness. Don't use complicated medical terms or try to tell your loved one too much all at once. Depending on the person's limitations and needs, you may want to use pictures, a video or a simply written handout.

4. Give the patient the details of the proposed treatment, test or surgery. Most important, explain what the experience will be like *from the patient's perspective.* What will it be like for the patient to experience the proposed treatment, test or surgery? Where will the test take place? Will the test hurt? Will it take all day? Will the patient

be left alone or can you stay with your loved one during the procedure? Will blood be drawn? Even if the patient can't give assent, your loved one should still be informed about what will be happening at the hospital or the doctor's office. A person with diminished capacity deserves to be treated with dignity, respect and compassion.

5. If the person says yes, be careful that the person isn't just saying that to make you happy. Make sure that the person really understands what is being discussed.

6. If the patient doesn't understand what you are talking about, then try again. If the person still can't understand, then you shouldn't use assent and you will need to make the full decision as if your loved one is developmentally zero to six years old.

Here's a real-life situation I had with my dad.

My dad's eyesight was getting worse, but I didn't realize how bad it had become until we went to the eye doctor. My dad couldn't see the big "E" on the eye chart.

My dad really wanted to have cataract surgery, but he was about twelve years old developmentally at the time, so he wasn't fully capable of giving his consent for the surgery. After the ophthalmologist fully explained the procedure to me and my dad, I asked my dad for his assent. "Dad, do you want to have the surgery?" I didn't make a big deal about it being only assent because it was important to help him keep his

Be sure to schedule regular eye and hearing exams for your loved one. Sometimes a patient's inability to participate in her life is due to a hidden physical limitation, rather than a mental limitation. You may discover that your loved one with diminished capacity improves when her hearing and vision improve.

self-respect. Since he understood what would happen to him with the surgery and he was comfortable with it, he said, "Yes, I want the surgery." Because this wasn't a life-or-death situation—cataract surgery is elective—my dad could have a strong voice in the decision. I was fine with his giving assent and I consented to the surgery. If there had been more risks involved or an increased chance of terrible side effects, I might have had to handle the situation differently. But this decision was safe for him to make and I knew I wasn't putting him in danger.

The Problem with Assent

Assent works great if the person gives you the answer you want to hear. But what if the person says, "No, I don't want to do that"? Have you ever asked a child if he wants ice cream and then have to tell him you are out of ice cream? The child probably began to cry or whine or yell.

Assent/dissent has this same issue. Your loved one is going to be very angry if you ask his or her opinion and then don't honor it. The patient can still communicate and voice concerns even if he or she doesn't have full capacity. Pediatricians are very careful about using assent correctly, because they don't want to break the trust they have with the child. Because pediatricians respect children, they will also apologize to the child when they have to do something against the will of the child.

The same concerns apply to you and your loved one. We always have to start this process from a place of respect and caring. You are in a long-term relationship with this person, so if you decide to ask your loved one for a yes or a no, then the person's decision should be honored. If your loved one really needs the surgery or procedure no matter what, then don't ask the question since you aren't going to be willing to accept no for an answer. Instead inform the person about what will be happening and give the necessary information to reassure and comfort your loved one.

Let's look at another example with my dad. What if my dad was having a different health issue and his doctor recommended a surgery that was a life-or-death decision? I would have said to my dad, "The doctor said you need to have this surgery," not "Dad, do you want to have this surgery?" I wouldn't have given him a false choice. Then I would have the doctor explain to my dad what would be happening to him and why, in a way my dad could understand. Even though my dad might not have a voice in this particular decision, he should still be treated with dignity. As the decision maker, your job includes protecting and caring for your loved one while making sure things go as well as can be expected.

Of course, let's not forget that I would have also considered what my dad would have wanted in this situation when he was fully capable. My dad would have said he wanted the surgery because he was still having a good life and wanted to have more time with his sisters, whom he loved. This is when I would have used the Substituted Judgment framework to make sure his values were being honored and his wishes were being respected. I would have also made sure that I was making a good medical decision for him and that surgery was the right treatment. As the decision maker, I would have asked more questions and worked with his doctors to make sure this was the right medical plan for my dad. As caregivers, we have to ask, "Is this the right medical treatment *and* is it something that my loved one would want?" The treatment has to be both *good for* the person and *wanted by* the person in order to be a good choice.

Does No Mean No?

What about those times when a treatment is not a life-or-death decision and the person gives you an answer that you don't agree with? Does no mean no? For now, it does. You can ask the person about the treatment at a later time, but be careful you aren't bullying your loved one into agreeing with you. Don't nag the person to change his or her mind just because you want to do things your way. Your loved one probably didn't like to be nagged when she had full capacity, and she won't like it now. She still has some capacity and some voice in her life. Your goal in this process is for the person to retain as much power in her life as possible for as long as possible. Keep in mind that it might be you in this situation someday. How would you want people to treat you? Wouldn't you want to be listened to and to have your choices respected?

If the assent/dissent process isn't working for you and your loved one, then a couple of things might be going wrong. You may be using the wrong tool or using it the wrong way. Perhaps you are letting the person have a voice in too important of a decision. Or perhaps the individual's mental condition is changing and you need to reevaluate whether or not the person should still participate in the process. It may be time to shift to the zero-to-six-year-old developmental age category. Or *you* may be the problem if you don't like what your loved one is choosing, and you are finding yourself in a power struggle as he is fighting to keep some control over his life. It might be some or all of these, but the main issue I see when assent fails is a problem with communication. We have to begin by asking ourselves, "Why isn't the person cooperating?"

Improving Communication When Asking for Assent

Many times people don't want to cooperate because they don't fully understand what we're talking about or how it will affect them. This happens a lot with those with dementia and Alzheimer's. They do not process the world as we see it and can become easily confused. Oftentimes, they won't agree to a particular test or treatment because they are afraid or uncertain. If a patient is afraid, then we have to find a new way to communicate to relieve her fears. Our goal is to help the person know what to expect. It may take repetition, a hands-on approach and concrete examples before a person with limited capacity can begin to understand her situation and possible treatments.

Another thing to keep in mind is that the patient may be experiencing symptoms that affect his decision making ability. These symptoms could be pain, side effects of medications, loss of hearing or sight, lack of sleep, an undiagnosed illness and grief, to name a few. Ask your loved one's doctor what can be done medically to relieve these symptoms to make it easier for him to participate in the process. And if the patient is grieving, get appropriate grief support for him. It is important to make the effort to find solutions to help the person stay engaged in life.

Here are some ways to help your loved one feel more comfortable. If the patient is struggling to understand what will happen during the treatment or test, do a practice run-through and show the person the room where the test will happen. Or find a book with pictures that will help your loved one understand what you are talking about. If the person with diminished capacity is afraid of being alone, you may want to introduce your loved one to the nurses who will be working that day. For my dad, we tape-recorded the doctor's explanations so that he could listen over and over again until he felt more comfortable. The trick is to find ways to give the information in a way that can be received by the specific individual. It is helpful to remember that when we teach a child to walk or to read, we are patient and allow the child the time he or she needs to learn the new skill. The same thing applies here. We need to be patient and to slow down the communication process. I know this will take time, but it is worth it to make the person feel more comfortable and empowered.

Be Careful When You Try This with Your Loved One

Since you don't want to put your loved one in a situation where he or she is given a false choice, before you begin to discuss a proposed treatment, test or surgery with him, make sure you have thought through the following questions before you tell the person he or she can have a voice. (For more specific help with making medical decisions, see chapter 10, "Making the Medical Decisions.")

- Is this an easy medical decision or is this a more serious situation?
- How risky is it to take this new medicine or have this test, treatment or surgery?
- How risky is it if my loved one does *not* have the treatment or surgery?

- Have I thought about what my loved one would want?
- Before you ask for your loved one's assent, ask yourself, "Is this a decision my loved one should have a voice in, or is this too important for me to take the chance that he or she might make the wrong choice?"

Fighting for Control

A few years ago, I was helping a father deal with his daughter who was newly diagnosed with bipolar disease. Life had become a battlefield in their house as the nineteen-year-old, who was just getting used to having her independence, didn't want to listen to her father. The father was trying to protect his daughter, but the more he tried to tighten his control over her, the more defiant the young woman became. Everything became a battle as the father tried to control every part of his daughter's day. He was trying too hard to do the right thing and thus made a huge mistake: He didn't need to control everything—just the things that were important for her safety.

One of the reasons that our loved ones argue with us is that people want to keep some control over their lives, especially when they feel as though they are out of control. We all want to have a voice. As people begin to lose their mental and/or physical abilities, they want to hold on tight to as much of their decision making power as possible.

When you say to your loved one, "You should do what the doctor told you to do," you sound as if you are trying to be the boss of this person. Yes, you are there to advocate, respect and protect your loved one, but that doesn't mean you have to control everything. If this is a person who still has some voice in his or her life, you will want to go back and use the Shared Decision Making concept of including the person to the level he or she is capable of. The father with the bipolar daughter could have picked his battles and allowed his daughter to keep some of her independence.

One way to help the person share in the decision making process and keep some control is to try "asking" instead of "telling": "What do you think about these options?" "What do you think would be the right thing to do?" "What would you suggest?" "Would you like some more time to think about this?" Then give the person the time and space to think about it.

If you find yourself in a conflict with your loved one, the first question to ask yourself is "Do I want my loved one to agree with me because this is the *right* thing to do or is it because I want things done *my way?*" I understand that this may be difficult to admit to yourself. We all have strong opinions about how things should be done, and we often think we know best. But be careful that you are not putting your opinions in front of the previously stated values of your loved one. Remember that, if possible, we are to respect and honor what the person would say he or she would want. If the person never liked to do something in the past, why would he or she want to do it now? Or if you find yourself pushing for something, even when the person has said no, ask yourself, "Am I respecting this person and his or her values? Why am I pushing so hard to get my way?" You might also want to check in with the decision making process and ask, "Am I using the right level of shared decision making with this person?" Even though it might seem easier to just take over the person's life, it is not a respectful or loving thing to do. If the roles were reversed, I don't think you would want someone to do that to you.

Babying Your Loved One

Sometimes I see people treating the person with diminished capacity as if he or she were a baby. This person is not a baby; he or she is an adult who needs your help and support. Yes, it is important to protect the person, but do not strip your loved one of his or her self-worth.

The other day, a woman was telling me about her dad's failing health. The father was still completely capable, but the daughter had taken over his life. Her dad had lost his voice. And everyone in the family started to overprotect him. When the grandkids visited, the adults would say, "Shush, don't bother your grandfather." But the grandfather loved interacting with his grandkids. He could still be their grandfather and he could still make a difference, even if he couldn't get out of bed anymore. He wasn't dead yet.

I encouraged the daughter to do her best to keep her dad included and valued within the family. I know when my aunt was dying, people would still come to her room and ask for her advice. She still mattered. I think this is one of the reasons she held on for so long. Her work wasn't done. Please help your loved one keep his or her dignity and value until the end.

You have an important role in making things better or worse for your loved one. You will need a lot of patience as you will have to explain things over and over again before the person will understand enough to participate in the decision. If you think about how you teach a child, you try to be consistent, set clear boundaries and follow through with the rules. If you are the kind of parent who says, "Stop that," but you don't really mean it, the child will know that you will give in and will keep testing you. The same things happen when grown-ups become childlike again. You have to set clear boundaries with rewards and punishments built in. You will need to give the person incentives to be more cooperative.

When the Person's Developmental Age Is Fourteen to Seventeen Years Old

So, what do you do if your loved one is developmentally fourteen to seventeen years old? This person may have full or almost full capacity, and if so, you should use autonomy and ask the patient directly for his or her consent or refusal. Remember from the Decision Making Framework that autonomy is used when the person has the capacity to determine what is right for his or her own body. If you think that the person who is developmentally fourteen to seventeen years old has full decisional capacity, then he or she should be allowed to make the decisions. (Remember that patients with capacity have the absolute right to make their own decisions, including the right to refuse life-saving treatments.) In getting informed consent, the doctor will check whether this person, young or old, can answer questions in a logical way. The doctor will ask the questions from the first core question to determine capacity.

If the time comes when your loved one has changed to a younger mental age, then you will need to go back and use the other tools you have learned. Always keep in mind that we are supposed to use the highest standard we can, based on the patient's ability to participate. Now we get to put all of these tools together into action.

7

How These Tools Work Together

As you begin putting the tools I've offered into action, it is very important that you use the right framework and the right tools or you may get a wrong answer. Let's begin by reviewing the four things you've learned so far in terms of a decision you face with your loved one.

1. Think back to the Decision Making Framework and determine if you will be using Substituted Judgment or the Best Interest Standard (p. 22).

2. Look at the Shared Decision Making Model to determine how much your loved one should be involved in the decision making process (p. 52).

3. Check with the Sliding Scale for Decision Making to decide how serious the decision is that you need to make and how you should proceed (p. 56).

4. Use the Assent Tool if your loved one's mental age is in the range of seven to thirteen and it is safe for the person to participate in the decision making process (p. 63).

If the person's mental age is in the range of zero to six, he or she will not be part of the decision making process. But you will still want to make sure the individual is told what will be happening and what to expect.

For those of you who would like to see how the core questions flow together in this decision making process, the 5 Core Questions Flowchart on pages 80 and 81 visually explains how these questions connect. This flowchart is your unofficial fifth tool, a map that you can use while making decisions. The flowchart is a useful tool to help you identify the right path for your loved one's situation. It has also been included to help the healthcare professional who is guiding caregivers through this process.

I know that many of you feel ready to begin to make decisions for your loved one. That's great. But some of you might want to practice a bit to make sure you understand how these tools work together. You don't want to start making decisions and then realize that you're using the wrong tool for the job. So let's try a couple of practice cases. I will give you a little help on the first one just in case you have any questions. Then you can try the rest yourself.

Testing Our New Knowledge

Case #1:

A thirty-five-year-old man was in a terrible car accident and now has a developmental age of nine. The patient used to be able to think for himself, and you know what he would have said to do in this life-or-death situation. The patient has an Advance Directive that indicates he wants his wife to make his decisions for him.

Answer the following questions:

- How important is this decision? (Life-or-death, important but not life-or-death, or not important)

- Which framework should I use? (Autonomy, Substituted Judgment or Best Interest Standard)

- What is the person's mental age? Should the person participate in the decision based on the age ranges in the Shared Decision Making Model? (0–6 years old, 7–13 years old or 14–17 years old)

- Who should be the decision maker?

Remember that the more important the decision, the higher the patient's mental age must be for him to participate.

Answer:

Because he has a developmental age of nine, you could use assent and allow the patient to participate. But since this is a life-or-death situation, you should inform him about what will be happening but not ask his opinion. Since you know what he

Figure 7.1:
5 Core Questions Flowchart

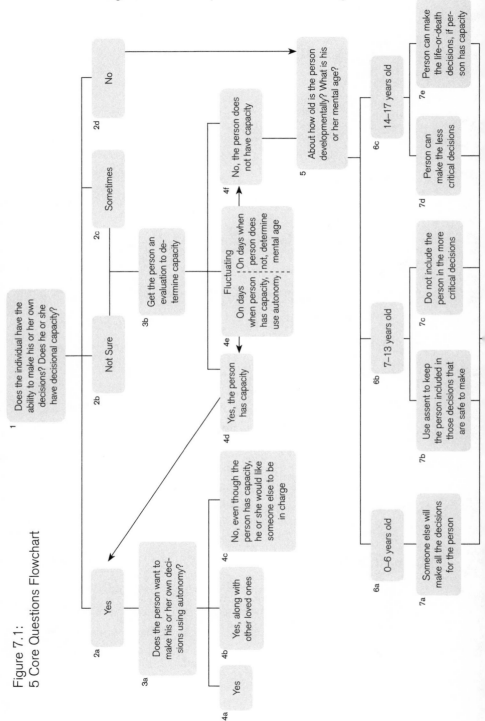

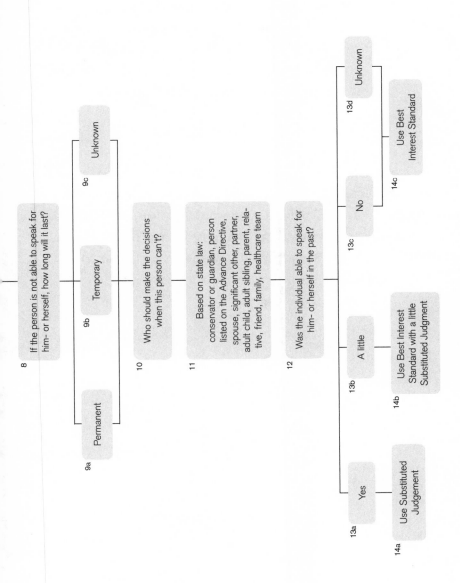

8 — If the person is not able to speak for him- or herself, how long will it last?

9a — Permanent
9b — Temporary
9c — Unknown

10 — Who should make the decisions when this person can't?

11 — Based on state law: conservator or guardian, person listed on the Advance Directive, spouse, significant other, partner, adult child, adult sibling, parent, relative, friend, family, healthcare team

12 — Was the individual able to speak for him- or herself in the past?

13a — Yes
13b — A little
13c — No
13d — Unknown

14a — Use Substituted Judgement
14b — Use Best Interest Standard with a little Substituted Judgment
14c — Use Best Interest Standard

would want, you will use Substituted Judgment and do what the patient would tell you to do. Because this patient had an Advance Directive, you should follow it—it represents his voice. His wife will be his decision maker. If he didn't have an Advance Directive, you would need to check the current laws in his state and decided who would be the appropriate decision maker.

Case #2:

A woman, age fifty-five, is developmentally delayed with a developmental age of one. She has never been able to express any preferences. A public conservator has been appointed by the county to make medical decisions for her. The decision to be made is about an elective surgery; the doctors indicated that they could wait to see if she can get better without it.

Answer the following questions:

- How important is this decision?
- Which framework should I use?
- What is the person's mental age? Should the person participate in the decision?
- Who should be the decision maker?

Answer:

With a developmental age of one, the patient will not be allowed to participate in the decision making process, even if it is a minor decision. Since this patient was never able to communicate any preferences, the conservator will have to use the Best Interest Standard. He should use the questions found in chapter 3, "The Best Interest Standard," as well as any questions that would help him from chapter 10, "Making the Medical Decisions." Because it is an elective surgery, the healthcare team and the public conservator—the decision maker in this case—should work together to decide if now is the right time for her to have the surgery or if it would be in her best interest to wait.

Case #3:

A sixty-three-year-old man with advancing Alzheimer's has a developmental age of eight. This patient used to be able to think for himself, but has now lost most of his ability to communicate. He can still communicate his basic preferences about what to eat or if he is in pain. He lives in a nursing facility and there is nobody to speak for him. The test the doctor wants him to have is important, but not life-or-death.

Answer the following questions:

- How important is this decision?
- Which framework should I use?
- Should the person participate in the decision? What is the person's mental age?
- Who should be the decision maker?

Answer:

This case is tricky, as things aren't as clear-cut as you would like. You will have to do the best you can and try to apply the tools appropriately.

If he is developmentally eight years old, he may be able to give his assent or dissent, depending on the situation. The problem is that his ability to communicate is slipping and his developmental age may be changing. If he really is eight years old mentally, you should try to find a different way to communicate with him. But you may need to reevaluate and perhaps adjust his developmental age to the zero-to-six-year-old age range.

The next problem is that although this isn't a life-or-death decision, it is important for him to get this test. If it is important enough, then you probably won't ask for assent/dissent. You will probably just inform him about what will be happening to him. But if it isn't that important, then you could try asking for his assent. This will be a judgment call. You will need the doctor's input to figure out how crucial this test really is for him.

Now you get to the biggest problem. There is nobody to speak for him and he doesn't have a conservator or guardian. The hospital may contact the court to have a conservator or guardian appointed. If not, the healthcare team will probably put together an advocacy team to make the decisions for him. This decision will depend on the rules in your state and the policy of the hospital.

If you are saying to yourself that there is still one piece missing, you're doing great. Are you going to use Substituted Judgment or Best Interest? This person used to be able to think and communicate for himself. But do you know what his preferences and values were in the past? Perhaps there is some indication in his medical records about what he would say regarding this type of medical situation. Perhaps he filled out an Advance Directive and there is a copy somewhere. Or perhaps the people where he lives can tell us a little something about what kind of person he used to be and what he used to value. Answering this question will take a bit of research, but it will be worth the effort if it helps you make the right choice for this patient.

Now that you have a better idea of how this all works together, it's time to try this with your own loved one's specific situation and details.

USING THE TOOLS
IN REAL LIFE

8

⁓

Applying Your New Skills to Real-Life Decisions

It is my hope that because of what you've learned so far, when you close this book and begin to make real-life decisions, it will be easier. I didn't say it would be easy, just easier. You will still struggle to make peace with the fact that you have had to take over your loved one's life. It may still be a battle to deal with an angry and demanding individual who hates it that he or she has lost control. And it won't be easy when you are crying alone at night, missing the person that your loved one used to be. I know how much I missed my energetic and capable dad.

Sometimes, it was really difficult to put my decisions into action for my dad, but what comforted me was that I knew I was doing the right thing. I knew that I had used the right tools and I was respecting and protecting him. I just had to be brave enough to take the necessary action. I think that as you become more confident in knowing you are doing the right thing for your loved one, you will find that you can speak with more authority when making the important decisions.

Here are the five core questions you have answered about your loved one.

1. Does the individual have the ability to make his or her own decisions? Does he or she have decisional capacity?
2. If the person is not able to speak for him- or herself, how long will it last?
3. Was the individual able to speak for him- or herself in the past?
4. Who should make the decisions when this person can't?
5. About how old is the person developmentally? What is his or her mental age?

Here are the three tools and the framework you can now use to make decisions.

1. The Decision Making Framework (pg. 22)
2. The Shared Decision Making Model (pg. 52)
3. The Sliding Scale for Decision Making (pg. 56)
4. The Assent Tool (pg. 63)

With these tools and information at hand, it's time to focus on your specific situation and the current condition of your loved one.

Action Questions

To simplify the process for you, I've combined all that you have learned into one set of questions. I call these your "Action Questions." Get out a piece of paper and write down the answers to the following Action Questions, based on what you know about your loved one. (In Appendix 3 I have given you a copy of these questions to photocopy and keep with you.)

1. What is the approximate mental age of the individual *today?*

2. Is this person able to make his or her own decisions?

3. If the person can't make his or her own decisions, will this lack of decision making ability continue or is it only temporary?

4. If the lack of capacity will only be for a short period of time, does this decision need to be made today or can I wait to see if he or she will regain the ability soon?

5. How important and serious is this decision?

6. Who should make the decisions while he or she has lost capacity?

7. Should this individual be involved in making this decision? If so, how much?

8. Was the person able to think and communicate in the past, and if so, was he or she fully capable or just partially capable?

9. Am I going to use Substituted Judgment or the Best Interest Standard?

10. What are the person's quality-of-life goals and what would he or she say in this situation?

> Beware of trying to rush through the process or skip questions. Remember that you have to use all the pieces of the puzzle to get to the right decision.

11. How can I keep the person included in ways that are safe for him or her to participate?

12. What other questions should I use from the checklists in this book?

Did you notice that these questions could apply even in everyday situations? They don't work just for healthcare decisions, but whenever you need to make decisions for your loved one. Anytime you need to figure out how much you should allow the person to participate in making life decisions, ask yourself the above Action Questions. If you are not sure or you need help because your decision making process isn't working, check back in with the prior strategies you have learned and let them guide you.

When it was time to move my dad from the nursing home into the dementia unit, I didn't ask his permission because his developmental age was about five years old. He needed to move because his needs weren't being met in the nursing home. Did I make it a big deal and point out all of the negatives about living in a dementia unit? Of course not. I tried to show him the positives and focused on the privileges he was going to have in this controlled environment. He would actually have more freedom than he did in his current environment. Did I let him pick which dementia facility he was going to move to? No. I evaluated which option was best for him and which one he could afford. I took care of the more serious decisions. But I tried to include him in the smaller decisions. Let me show you how I did this.

The next time I visited, I told him about the new place. I then took him to visit the place ahead of time so that he could be comfortable with the move. When we got there I said, "This is where you will be living." I didn't ask him if he would like to live there. Then I asked him, "Do you want to pick which room you will get?" He was thrilled. We looked at three different rooms and he picked the one he wanted. He grinned the rest of the day and kept saying, "Viki, I got a really good room. That room was better than all the rest." He got to make the decision that was safe for him to make. The next decision he got to make was about his personal belongings. He was going to be able to have more of his personal belongings in the dementia unit, so I had him tell me what he wanted me to move into his new room. Of course, I brought the necessary bath chair and other safety devices, but he got to choose the other items. Again, I included him as much as possible in those decisions that were safe for him to make.

Don't forget that this is a new process for you and that it may take some time to get comfortable doing it. Decision making will get easier and faster as you use the process more and more. And eventually, you won't even need to go through the process of answering the Action Questions—you will just know what to do. To help you down that path, I'm going to walk you through some of the common decisions people have to make for those in their care.

Decision: Starting a New Medication

The doctor wants to start your loved one on a new medication. Should you have the person take the medicine? The first step is to review your answers to the Action Questions and apply them to this situation.

As you make this decision, you will you need to ask more medical questions. What are the risks with this new medication? What are the benefits? Why does the doctor want to use this medicine and not try something else? Is it covered by your loved one's insurance? Would your loved one say that he would want to take this medicine? If you need more information, you can use the questions in chapter 10, "Making the Medical Decisions."

Decision: Taking the Car Keys Away

You just got a call that your loved one has been found driving on the wrong side of the road and she seems confused. Should you take her car keys away? Apply your answers to the Action Questions to this situation.

You will want to find out why the person was driving on the wrong side of the road. Was she having a momentary problem because she had just started a new medication, or is something more serious and long lasting going on? You will probably need to get a medical evaluation to answer this question. Your loved one may also need to be evaluated by a geriatric driving specialist. For now though, you will need to take away the keys because this is a life-or-death situation. This option may be necessary only for a short period of time, but you cannot take a chance with the life of your loved one and all the other people on the road. You can't allow her to keep driving while you find out the answers. If the problem can be corrected, then she can regain her driving privileges. If not, the keys should be taken away permanently.

When and How to Take the Car Keys Away

Dear Viki,

My grandfather is losing his memory. The other day he got in a minor accident and couldn't or wouldn't tell the police where he lived or who to call. Nobody else in the family seems to recognize there is a problem, but I do. I don't want to be the one to do it, but should I take away my grandfather's car keys?

My answer:

I understand what you are going through because I had to take away my dad's keys. He was getting more and more confused and forgetful. I was lucky because I took away his keys before he hurt himself or someone else. But many people aren't that lucky. Their loved one kills someone by accident and the whole family is devastated. Even if others aren't seeing what you see, you need to do the right thing.

So the answer to your question is *yes*. And do it now. You should take away his keys today before anything worse happens. What helped me make the decision for my dad was realizing that I was protecting him from himself. I had noticed that his behavior was getting worse, but I didn't want to face it. I wanted to believe that things weren't that bad. But they were. I knew that if he drove again and hurt someone, it would be my fault because now that I knew there was a problem, I would be responsible. I couldn't live with myself if someone died because I wasn't brave enough to do the right thing.

I am not saying this will be easy. My dad hated that I took away his keys. And I had to go through the whole house to find all the copies of the keys. I realized when I found fifteen copies of the keys that he had been forgetting where he kept his keys and kept getting copies made. Another solution families choose is to disable the vehicle so the person can't start the car even if there are more keys hidden in the house. Eventually my dad got rid of his car so he didn't have to be reminded of his loss.

And yes, it will be a loss. And yes, your grandfather will be angry and sad. He should be upset. This is the moment when he will realize that he has lost control over his life. He is experiencing not only the loss of driving but also the loss of his independence. He now has to depend on you. I know that someday when my niece or nephew takes away my car keys, I am going to be so disappointed. It will be a terrible loss, but hopefully I will remember that my family is protecting me and loving me. I hope that one of them has the courage to do the right thing, even if doing the right thing is difficult. If you don't have the courage, ask the doctor to tell your grandfather that he can no longer drive.

When the time comes, it is a good idea to sit with your grandfather and let him speak his mind. All you have to do is listen. Don't defend yourself. Don't defend the doctor. Just listen. As you hear his words, think about the day when you will lose your driving privileges, and find compassion for him.

One technique you can use is active listening. With active listening you repeat back the words and the emotions you are hearing. For example, when your grandfather says, "I am so mad at you for telling the doctor that I shouldn't be driving anymore," you can say, "I understand that you're really mad at me, Grandpa, and you wish I hadn't told the doctor." Your natural instinct will be to defend yourself or to explain the reasons you did what you did. Try not to do this. Instead, remember that this conversation is not about facts, it is about emotions. Just hear his heart and allow him to experience his feelings. Say supportive and acknowledging things like: "I know you are really angry right now, Grandpa. I would be too." "You have a right to be angry." "I am so sorry that you can't drive anymore." "I would be angry too if I couldn't drive anymore." Don't tell him he shouldn't feel what he feels. He is entitled to his emotions.

As he feels heard, he will calm down, although it may take a while. It may even take a number of conversations, so don't be surprised or upset if it does. Don't you sometimes have to vent more than once about something you are dealing with in your life? Just accept that this is part of the healing process. Hopefully over time, he will come to terms with this loss and move on in his life. But don't expect him to be happy about losing the ability to drive. It will always be a disappointment.

Decision: Moving to a Care Facility or Group Home

It may be time to move your loved one into some kind of long-term care facility or group home. You will have to figure out which places can meet the needs of your loved one, which places have a bed or room available, and which places you can afford. This is a complex decision. You will have some research to do. Once you have more information, then you can figure out if your loved one should be a part of this decision and if so, how much? Don't forget to use the Action Questions so that you don't forget any of the decision making steps.

If the individual can make her own decisions, then this decision isn't yours to make. If the person is still safe at home, wants to stay at home and can afford it, then respect your loved one's autonomy and wishes. But if this person is putting herself at risk because it is now dangerous for her to live by herself, then you may have to step in to protect her. Keep in mind that a person with full decisional capacity has the right to make bad decisions, including the decision to live where it isn't safe. But the fact that this person may not recognize the danger she is in may mean your loved one is beginning to lose her capacity. You will need to get a medical evaluation of your loved one's mental and physical condition.

You will probably need a team of people to help you manage this situation. Begin by talking to your loved one's doctors, the hospital's social worker, and a local geriatric care manager or patient advocate. You can also evaluate the different options that are available. Perhaps you can make the house safer. Perhaps you can get someone to help in the home. Or perhaps it really is time for the individual to move to a care facility. There are professionals in the community who can address the housing safety issue and can give you guidance. You may need to contact Adult Protective Services to help you protect your loved one if the situation falls under elder abuse laws or disability protection laws.

Decision: A Life-or-Death Medical Decision

Your loved one's doctor says that your loved one has to have surgery to save her life. Should you agree to the surgery and sign the consent form? Should your loved one be included in the decision?

Unless your loved one has almost full capacity, you are probably going to make this decision because it is life-or-death. Be careful, though, that you don't just say yes because it is life-or-death. Not only must you evaluate the medical decision, you must also consider what your loved one would say about this decision and how it will affect her long-term quality of life. Ask yourself, "If the patient were able to wake up and understand what is going on, what would she say should be done?" If the person would say yes, then make sure you choose the right doctor and hospital for this type of surgery. (Use the questions in chapter 10, "Making the Medical Decisions.")

If your loved one would say no, then the answer is no. People are allowed to say no even to treatments that would save their lives. If this is the case, then you will need to get the support of the hospital's social worker, a chaplain and/or your family and friends. This is when honoring your loved one becomes very painful for the decision maker. Saying no when you wish your loved one would say yes creates grief and moral distress.

The next chapter will discuss how our emotions may be affecting our decision making process.

9

*

When Our Hearts
Get in the Way

So far, I have been giving you very practical advice. I now want
to change directions and talk about when your heart gets in the
way of good decision making. Whether you have had a difficult
relationship with this person or this person is the love of your
life, your emotions will affect your ability to think clearly and
to come up with a good plan. No matter what, your reaction
to this person and the situation, good or bad, will be affecting
your judgment. That's okay. You are human and you are not
the only caregiver who has had these strong emotions. I know
that I have had to stop and have a good cry or to take a walk
to calm down or clear my head before I could make good decisions about difficult situations with my dad.

Emotions become a danger when we pretend they aren't affecting us or we ignore them altogether. It is much better to stop and acknowledge what we are feeling. When we do this, we can put the emotion into perspective and realize the role our emotional reaction is having in our decision making process. Emotions aren't bad unless they are clouding your judgment or leading you to make the wrong decision. One of the best ways I know to deal with this obstacle is to slow down and take the time to feel what you are feeling. When you are ready, put the emotion aside and start thinking again. This isn't easy, but just becoming aware of this issue will help you make clearer and more appropriate decisions.

The following topics are just a few of the many ways our emotions play a role in our interactions with our loved ones.

Choosing the Least Worst Option

As you begin your decision making journey, I want to acknowledge that sometimes we have to choose between a bad option and a really bad option. What often helps is realizing that sometimes we have to pick the "least worst option." What does this mean? It means you don't always get to use a "good answer" or a "good choice" when making a decision. The only choice is to pick the least terrible option, because that is the best option available. I know this is horrible, but we have to make peace with this dilemma. Of course, we first have to work hard to determine if there are better options available, asking other people for help as we research the choices. But sometimes it will come down to a decision that will never feel right or good. All you can do is to do the best you can and pick the least worst option.

The Promises We Can't Keep

The other day, a man told me that he didn't know what to do. He had promised his mom that he would never put her in a nursing home. But now, because of her Alzheimer's, she needed more care than he could provide. He didn't want to break his promise but he couldn't protect her from herself. Just this week, she had started a fire in the kitchen.

This situation can be so painful. We all want to do the right thing, but sometimes it becomes impossible. I explained to the man that even though he had made a promise, he couldn't stand by and let his mom be in harm's way. He hadn't known when he made that promise what was to come.

I encouraged him to do what he could to keep her at home. Perhaps he could hire more help or make the house safer. But if those options didn't work, he had to forgive himself and do the right thing and find a good care facility. This doesn't mean he won't feel badly about going back on his word. This is the hard road of caregiving.

Reconnecting with Your Loved One—The Pajama Story

My friend told me the most touching story the other day.

A sweet lady was a devoted and loving wife to her dying husband for over forty-five years. She did everything for him at home, but as the end neared, she had to admit her husband to an inpatient hospice facility so that he could get the help he needed to manage his symptoms. This ended up being the best situation—for both of them. Because there were other people available to take over the care of her husband, she was finally free to put on her pajamas and crawl into bed beside him. She spent the last three days before he died with him as his wife, not as his caregiver. It was the first time in months that she could stop and reconnect with the love of her life.

I cried when I heard this. It is so easy to get caught up in the work and responsibility of caregiving and miss the opportunity to enjoy your loved one while you still have him with you. This person is not a body to be turned or fed or cleaned, but the person you love. We only have so many days with the people we value, so take a moment every day or as often as you can to enjoy your time together, no matter where you are in the caregiving process. Start now. Put on your pajamas and remember why you have devoted yourself to this person. These are precious moments not to be wasted.

Near the end of my dad's life, we were waiting at the doctor's office and there was music playing. I asked my dad to dance. He loved to ballroom dance, and although he could barely stand, he and I had a dance in the middle of the waiting room. I took an everyday moment and made it special. We both treasured it, as that was the last time he was able to stand up long enough to dance. He quickly declined after that and we never danced again.

Are You Experiencing "Care-grieving"?

You are normal if you are experiencing what I call "care-grieving"—the grief that comes with caring for and caring about another person. Not only is caregiving exhausting, overwhelming, frustrating and emotionally draining, it is also associated with profound grief.

So why might you be care-grieving?

You may be grieving because your loved one isn't the person she used to be. You used to look to your loved one to support and nurture you, and now that aspect of your relationship is gone. Your loved one may still be physically alive, but the person you knew is no longer with you.

Your grief may be over the dramatic changes in your life. Maybe you had to quit work. Maybe you don't have time for yourself anymore. Maybe you know that you aren't being as good of a parent to your own kids as you used to be. Maybe you have to pay your loved one's bills. All of these changes create a sense of loss. It doesn't mean you're a bad person if you feel angry or sad. You are normal and your grief is normal.

You may also be care-grieving because you realize that your loved one is going to die, possibly soon. This is called *anticipatory grief* because we anticipate the loss and begin grieving before that loss is a reality. Sometimes this loss comes along slowly and sometimes it rushes toward us. Either way, it is painful and difficult. Unfortunately, oftentimes nobody will talk to you about this. People will tell you to stop worrying or to put on a happy face. But this grief is real and normal. Each day, as you witness the changes in your loved one's physical and mental abilities, your grief grows. Try to find somebody that you can talk to about your anticipatory grief.

Maybe your grief is over your own mortality. Maybe you have realized that when your parents die, it will be your turn next. The first time someone told me I was now an orphan after both of my parents had died, I hated it. It reminded me of how much I had lost and that I was of the next generation in line to die.

There are many other ways you may be care-grieving. You may feel like you're missing out on life. Your health may be deteriorating. You may want to run and hide. You may wish your loved one would just go ahead and die. Oops. Was I supposed to say that aloud? Probably not, but I know people have whispered it to me, and they were good, loving, amazing children of aging parents. Care-grieving can become so overwhelming that it creates in us a desperation and a need to survive. It's not that we wish our loved one was gone, we just wish our pain was gone. Those who have said it to me continued to give and to love and to support their loved ones, but they needed to reach out for support for themselves as well.

Ultimately, you can't get around grief. You have to get through it. You have to experience it and allow the emotions to be felt and heard. You need to talk about it with people who can help you. This may be your family, but often we have to look to outsiders for this support, as our family members may be grieving too. Please reach out for support from your friends, your extended family and your religious community. You can also get help from local support groups, from online forums and chat rooms and from anyone else who may be willing to listen. If it is getting to be too much, seek professional help.

Care-grieving is normal, but ongoing suffering is not. Please get the help you need.

Caregiver Burnout—Getting the Support You Need

If you are in caregiver burnout, you won't be able to make good decisions. I was the caregiver for a number of family members for many, many years. Sometimes I could manage just fine. But at other times I felt overwhelmed and unappreciated. Even when I knew what to do, I was still exhausted and worried all the time. All I wanted to do was to crawl into bed and just sleep. Even though I wanted to take care of the seniors in my life, sometimes it all became too much.

I admire professionals who take care of those who are disabled, sick or dying every day. But I also know it comes at a cost to the person doing the caregiving. So, let's talk about the signs of caregiver stress and then

Because caregiving can be so fatiguing, you probably have days when you can't keep track of everything that needs to be done. I know that the only things that kept me sane when I was taking care of multiple relatives were my to-do lists. To help you maintain control of all the information and duties coming at you, you may want to keep a piece of paper or a notebook nearby. When you are on the phone, write down whom you are talking to, what was said, the time and date of the call, and other questions or thoughts you have during the call. Keep a list of questions you need to ask the doctor or other calls you have to make.

discuss ways you can ask for help. (Help is out there, even if it doesn't come from your family.)

Here are just some of the signs of caregiver stress and burn-out: feeling physically exhausted, emotionally overwhelmed, anxious, hopeless, angry, depressed, isolated, mentally drained, lonely and frustrated. You may be too tired to make the effort to do the things you used to do for yourself or your loved one. You might be getting ill yourself. You may feel as though nobody is listening to your concerns. You may want to lash out at your co-workers or your friends and family.

Why do caregivers burn out? Here are a few reasons.

- Caregivers may not be able to sleep because their loved ones are up all night.
- Caregivers may not have the necessary training to offer the care that is needed.
- Caregivers may be physically doing more than they can.
- Caregivers may have to quit their jobs to stay home with their loved ones.
- Caregivers may go bankrupt because of increasing expenses.
- Caregivers may feel guilty if they take time out for themselves.
- Caregivers may feel that they should be strong and not need any help.
- And caregivers usually don't ask for help.

Unfortunately, by the time you need extra help, you may be too tired, emotionally fatigued or depressed to ask for it. You have to get a support team in place when you begin caregiving so that you don't get to your breaking point. Start planning ahead of time, before you need the help.

There are people and organizations trained to help people in distress. The first person to ask is the patient's primary doctor. The doctor won't be able to send in someone to take over for you, but he or she may be able to order a visiting nurse, medical equipment or to help you find a person to help. You can also hire a geriatric care manager or a patient advocate—people who can help design and put into place a plan to get you the help you need. This is especially helpful if you live a significant distance away from your loved one. Another person you can turn to is your local hospital's social worker, who already knows the resources available in your town and can give you a list of people you could call. Organizations such as Meals on Wheels, Dial-a-Ride, religious organizations and your local senior center can help and are usually free. Illness- or condition-specific organizations, such as the Alzheimer's Association, the American Heart Association, the American Stroke Association, the Brain Injury Association of America, the National Alliance on Mental Illness and the Hospice Foundation of America, can provide support and information.

Another great option to consider is an adult day care facility. Once your loved one gets used to the new place, she will enjoy getting out and interacting with others and you will enjoy the break. (And your loved one might enjoy a break from you too.) There may also be night care available in your community so that you can get a good night's sleep.

You may also want to look into online support groups, local support groups, and individual and group therapy options. There are also support groups available for your loved one. You don't have to be the only person giving your loved one comfort and support. Ask for help for your loved one and for yourself.

You don't have to feel alone or be alone with the stressors you are facing. But people won't know you need help unless you tell them. Speak up and speak out to get what you and your loved one needs. And don't forget to give yourself credit for all that you are already doing. You don't have to be a superhero—you already are an everyday hero.

Protecting the Caregiver

Before we continue on, I would like to stop and give you a gift that you can use to protect yourself. One of the best things you can do for yourself is to consider completing your own Advance Directive. You can't fill out an Advance Directive for someone who has lost capacity, but you can fill out your own. When you have an Advance Directive, it will empower your own decision maker to know and respect your wishes. It will also help the doctors to know what to do for you. I encourage you to think about protecting the people you care about so that in the future, your family or friends won't be in the position you are in right now and not know what to do. For more information, "An Insider's Guide to Filling Out Your Advance Directive" can be found in Appendix 2. You'll understand how important an Advance Directive can be as you read the following chapters on making medical decisions for your loved one.

One other thing you might consider doing is getting a long-term care insurance policy, which is an insurance policy that goes into effect when you become significantly disabled and need long-term care. Your loved one probably does not qualify, but *you* can still get the financial protection that a long-term care policy provides. My dad had a policy and each month, the insurance company sent a check that covered his expenses in the dementia unit. After I saw how much this insurance saved my dad's financial health, I made sure that I got a policy too. If you are going to buy this kind of insurance, please take the time to do the necessary research to make sure you are making a good decision.

Seeing It from Your Loved One's Perspective

Throughout this book, I have reminded you to look at these decisions through your loved one's eyes and to keep the person included as much as possible when appropriate. I would like to stop for a minute and ask you to really feel what it is like for this individual with diminished capacity. It is time for you to trade places with the person you are caring for and to consider the world from his or her perspective.

Imagine what it would feel like to have someone else be in charge of your life. You don't get to decide where you are going, how you will get there or what will happen when you arrive. You have to do things on someone else's schedule now.

How would it feel to know that you are losing your mind? You are still the same person, but somehow different. You try to remember things, but you know you keep forgetting. You try to speak but the words aren't there. You can't do the things you used to do and you feel helpless all the time. Without your voice, you feel as though you no longer exist. You are at the mercy of others whether you like it or not.

People treat you differently. They treat you like a child and don't take you seriously. They speak in a sing-song voice as they would with a baby. When you do talk, people don't listen or respect what you say. People talk as if you are not even in the room. You feel invisible. Just once, you would like to be *you* again.

Maybe you are in the midst of terrible grief. All of these losses are overwhelming, but nobody is willing to talk to you about your sadness. You wish that someone would listen to your complaints and let you cry about what you are going through.

You are no longer able to do things physically; you need help with the simplest of tasks. You have to wait until someone comes to help you to the bathroom, and sometimes while you are waiting, you can't hold it any longer and you have to use your diaper. Oh my goodness. You are wearing diapers.

And perhaps you can't even feed yourself without someone's help. Or maybe you can't swallow and now you are fed through a tube. What would it be like to never taste food again?

I don't know about you, but I would feel angry, frustrated, embarrassed, sad, isolated, lonely, depressed, vulnerable and out of control.

Write down how you would feel if you had to cope with what your loved one is experiencing. Then write down what you think it is like for your loved one to be in this situation. If you can, ask the person directly what is the most difficult part of experiencing this new condition. It is okay to admit to your loved one that the situation is hard and that everybody is struggling. Too often, we pretend that nothing is wrong, and this isolates us—and our loved ones even more. Instead, talk about how you are each coping. Allow the person to share his emotions, even the loud and scary emotions. Be still and listen with your full attention. Turn off the phone and the television. Be present with your loved one's suffering. When you listen, you help the person heal.

Ask your loved one what he or she would like to have happen. Include the person in every way you can think of so she can retain some sense of control and power. This is one of the greatest gifts you can give your loved one. And then, each time you have to make a decision for your loved one or to talk about life choices, remember to start from his or her perspective.

I know this journey is difficult for you, the caregiver, but keep in mind how difficult it is for your loved one. Perhaps you can be a little more patient or a little more respectful. Maybe before you lash out in frustration with the person you are caring for, you can stop, catch your breath and try to be more understanding, compassionate and kind. I know you are human and you can't be nice all the time. I know I have been frustrated and less than loving at times when taking care of my family members. But I also know we can strive to be better— not perfect, but better. It's not easy, but we can choose to do a little better every day. Now, let's get back to work and learn how to make better medical decisions.

10

Making the Medical Decisions

In chapter 8, I gave you Action Questions to help you with the decision making process. Those questions are an important first step. But what happens when you are responsible for making complicated medical decisions for your loved one? The Action Questions aren't enough.

This chapter and the next two will give you a whole new way of looking at how medical decisions should be made. Most of the patients I help will make an instant medical decision after getting just one or two pieces of information from a doctor. If making a quick decision works for you in your own life, then that is okay with me. But this book is about making decisions for other people. You have to take this responsibility seriously and take the time to ask enough questions to feel confident that you're making the right decisions.

One of the biggest obstacles I see in healthcare today is the pressure of time. The healthcare team may be overworked and behind schedule. Even though you may feel the pressure to hurry up and make the decision, you usually have enough time to stop and determine what questions to ask, what you should consider and what would be the right thing to do. Unless it is an emergency, ask the doctor for a little bit of time to think through the treatment options and to apply the answers from your Action Questions.

Balancing the Benefits and the Risks

To slow down the process and to give you time to think, you can write down the benefits and the risks or burdens of the options that are available. When doctors are designing the right medical treatment plan for your loved one, they ask, "Do the benefits outweigh the burdens and risks?" If you aren't familiar with this type of decision making model, think about the decision like an old-fashioned scale. On one side of the scale are the benefits and on the other side are the burdens and risks. For each decision, you should determine which option will give you the best results with the fewest risks and side effects.

Let's try this example. A twenty-nine-year-old veteran has recently returned home with a brain injury and needs a non–life-or-death surgery. The doctors think that this surgery will help to move along the healing process for him. Right now, this wounded warrior is unable to participate in decision making, so the decision rests with his wife. What should she decide?

Benefits/Good

- 60% chance that he will recover more mental capacity

Burdens/Risks/Bad

- 40% chance that it won't work
- The surgery could make him worse
- Risk of death during the surgery
- Long and difficult recovery process

I don't know what his wife will decide, because she doesn't have enough information yet. There are many questions that she will need to ask. She will need more specific information about the surgery and the recovery process. As his wife collects more information and asks more questions, she should put the information she learns on the benefit or the burden side of the scale. It doesn't matter how many items or how much information she puts on the scale, what matters is the importance of each item. In addition to the benefits and risks, she must also consider what her husband would want if he could speak for himself. Her husband is a brave man and he would be willing to take the chance in spite of the risks. She also knows he will be able to do the hard work of recovering. Ultimately, it comes back to what the patient would say in this situation once he had heard all the information. And if he would say yes, his wife should say yes for him.

One thing I would like to caution you about is that some doctors will focus only on the medical aspects of the decision. While this is a medical decision, I believe that you can't reach a good decision without considering the whole context of the person's life. This is why I would encourage you to use at least some of the questions from the lists in this chapter and the next two chapters—questions about medical issues, financial issues, religious or spiritual concerns, cultural concerns, personal values and quality-of-life goals. Please do not be overwhelmed by the number of questions—many of them may not apply to you. I wanted to be as complete as possible because different people and families and communities have different concerns. Use the questions that relate to your loved one's situation or write your own questions, as you know best what else might be relevant.

Another problem I see is that people will get caught up in the day-to-day details of the patient's condition and forget to ask about the long-term picture. So when the doctor tells you about the latest lab or X-ray results, make sure you ask how this new information fits in with the bigger picture of the patient's health. Ask the doctor what is expected in the long term so that you can make the right short-term decisions along the way.

Some people make the mistake of not asking enough questions or asking the wrong questions. If you aren't sure where to start, you might want to ask others what they would want to know if they were in this same type of situation. Ask the professionals you are working with, "What do other people ask in this situation?" and "What else am I forgetting to ask?" You may also need to get second opinions from other healthcare professionals and do your own research as you go through these questions. Make sure you are using trusted websites, as not everything on the Internet is true. The doctor can help you figure out which websites are good to use.

And don't forget to consider your loved one's wishes. To gather information about what your loved one would want, you may need to talk to other family members and friends of your loved one—people he may have talked to about these issues.

This research will take some time, but unless it is an emergency, you should think about the questions in these next chapters so that you can make a good decision. You will feel better knowing that you took the time to stop and think so you could do right by your loved one.

Asking Good Medical Questions

When you are talking to your loved one's doctor, bring your list of questions, paper to write down the answers and a tape recorder if the doctor will allow it. Ask all of the questions you need to ask until you have the information needed to make a good, informed decision.

If your list of questions is very long, you may have to go back for a second appointment because doctors only have so much time per appointment. The questions below are grouped into subgroups to make it easier for you to pick and choose the ones that will help you deal with the current medical situation.

> **Informed Consent or Informed Refusal:** A doctor has to give a patient or a decision maker enough information so that a good, informed decision can be made regarding the treatment options.

Medical Questions

The following questions can be downloaded from my website, TheCaregiversPath.com.

Time:

- Is this an emergency, or is there time to think about what should be done?
- If it is not an emergency, how long do we have to make a decision?

Diagnosis or condition:

- What do you call what the patient has?
- How bad is the patient's condition?
- How many other things are going wrong with the patient's body?
- Are those other things fixable?

Available treatment options:

- Is this the first time I have had to make decisions about this illness or condition, or has it been going on a long time?
- What worked in the past?
- Is that still an available option?
- What are the other available options?
- What is the proposed treatment, surgery or test?
- Who will perform the treatment, surgery or test?
- How realistic is it that the proposed plan will work?

- Is the proposed treatment standard or is it experimental?
- How many times has the doctor done this procedure?
- What is the doctor's success rate?
- What has the doctor's success rate been with patients in a similar condition?
- Is there anything I can do to increase my loved one's chances of a good outcome?

Alternatives:

- What alternatives are available?
- What will happen if nothing is done?
- What will happen if we wait until later?
- Why now and not later?

Possible side effects:

- What are the possible risks and side effects?
- How often do the side effects really occur?
- What steps will be taken to minimize the risks of the treatment?

Suffering:

- How much is my loved one suffering now?
- How much will the patient suffer if he or she *does not* have this treatment?
- How much will the patient suffer if he or she *does* have this treatment?
- What can be done to prevent or decrease the suffering?

Benefits of the treatment:

- Will the treatment help the person regain or improve his or her mental function?
- Will the treatment help the person regain or improve his or her physical function?
- Do the benefits of the treatment outweigh the risks and burdens?
- Will the proposed treatment extend the patient's life, and for how long?
- What is the patient's life expectancy without the treatment?
- Will the proposed treatment improve the quality of the patient's life or only increase the length of life?

The patient's perspective:

- Would the patient want to have this treatment, surgery or test?
- Does this treatment plan fit in with the patient's quality-of-life goals?
- Does this treatment make sense in the context of this particular patient's life?
- What kind of condition will the patient be in afterward?
- What kind of life will the patient have after he or she is discharged from the hospital?

Other concerns:

- What do I *not* want to believe about what the doctor is saying?

- What do the different doctors say that is conflicting?
- Can I ask for a family conference so the doctors can explain why they disagree with each other?
- What am I confused about, and what questions do I need answered before I can decide?
- Do I need to get a second opinion to get more options or information?
- Am I reading information on the Internet from trusted sources? (If not, you need to ask the doctor which sites are recommended.)
- What do other people ask in this situation?
- What else am I forgetting to ask?

Possible restrictions:

- Are there hospital restrictions that limit what options are available here (religious restrictions, location restrictions, equipment restrictions, technical ability restrictions or the availability of specialists)?
- Are there laws that I need to be aware of in this situation? (Ask a social worker if there are any laws in your state that limit what a decision maker is allowed to agree to for the patient.)

After the treatment (or nontreatment):

Make sure to follow up to see how the patient is reacting to the treatment. Your job is not done as long as the person is receiving medical care. You have to keep an eye on how the person's health is changing over time.

- Is the patient doing better?
- Did the treatment help?
- Is the treatment making the patient worse?
- If the patient is not receiving the treatment, how is the person doing without the proposed treatment?
- Do I need to change my mind and work with the doctors to create a new plan?

As you use these questions, you will sometimes find it easy to make decisions because the benefits are numerous and the risks or burdens are so few that it makes obvious sense to go forward with the recommended treatment plan. But in those situations that aren't as clear-cut, I think you will find these questions to be most helpful. Using these questions will also help you when you are in a conflict with either the healthcare team or other family members who are helping with the decision.

Don't be afraid to keep asking the doctor for more information until you have what you need. But remember that the doctor may have other patients in a crisis in the hospital. So be patient if the doctor can't stay and answer all of your questions right away. Ask the doctor when he will return so you can finish your conversation. Be polite and be persistent.

When the Plan Doesn't Work or Can't Work

You may find that you made the best medical decision you could and then the plan didn't work. When this happens, it is important to reconsider the treatment plan. Otherwise, you're driving down the wrong road: You can keep driving and driving, but you will never get to where you are going. You need to stop, ask for new directions and then start down a new path.

You may also need to modify your expectations when things don't work. Sometimes we are so desperate for the plan to work that we can't bear to see the truth when the plan fails. You are not helping your loved one by continuing treatments that don't work. You are only subjecting the patient to needless side effects and increased suffering.

One thing that doctors may want to do is to try a time-limited trial of a proposed treatment option. "Let's try it for a few days or for a little while and see how it goes." This is a really great option. After the set time expires, you can check to see if the decision is working. If it is not working, go back through the decision making process and make a better decision based on the new information about the patient's changing condition. Don't be stubborn and keep driving your loved one in the wrong direction. Take this as an opportunity to turn around and get it right.

Now let's move on and look at some of the other issues you might want to consider when making these decisions.

11

⌒

Other Questions to Consider When Making Medical Decisions

Your loved one's doctor will talk to you about the medical aspects of any health-related decision. But that doesn't mean that you are limited to thinking only about medicine. It may be important to consider the financial costs associated with the treatment plan, if the patient's religion should play a role in the decision and whether there are cultural issues that come into play. These next questions are for you to use when thinking about the overall picture of your loved one's life.

It would be nice for the decision to be as simple as asking, "Will the treatment work and what are the side effects?" But life isn't that simple. What if you were about to make a medical decision that allowed something to be done to the person's body that was forbidden by the person's culture or religion? You might have chosen a certain treatment to save her life, but because the patient received that treatment, she will no longer be able to move on to the hereafter. Yes, the medical decision was a good one, but how the decision will affect the person's life, based on her personal belief system, was not.

If the person you are making decisions for is very religious, then it would be good to find out if there are any religious rules or values that you should consider in your decision making. I know that when I work with my hospice patients, it is important to know if there are certain rites or blessings that have to be performed before the patient's death. I don't have to agree with what the person wants, but if I am the caregiver, then I need to do what I can to make sure the person's religion or culture is respected. I will need to call in the appropriate religious leader to take care of the spiritual needs of this person. If the person is not religious or spiritual, then you will need to respect this and leave religion out of the decision making process.

For most people, the financial costs of the medical treatment will need to be considered or you may be putting the person in financial danger. You may be in charge of making only the healthcare decisions, but you should make sure that you or somebody else checks with the insurance company to find out whether or not it will pay for the treatment and to get the proper authorizations. Don't let a simple mistake like forgetting to call the insurance company to let them know that your loved one was admitted to the hospital put your loved one in financial distress. Making decisions without using the financial questions could bankrupt your loved one. Our goal of protecting the person should include protecting his or her wallet.

Financial Questions

The following questions can be downloaded from my website, TheCaregiversPath.com.

Patient finances:

- Does the patient have enough money to pay the doctors, the hospital, the X-ray department, the laboratory and the other medical bills?
- If not, can the patient get the money or is this impossible?
- Can the patient afford the medications both now and for the long term?

Cost of treatment:

- Can I get an estimate of the costs before I decide?
- Does this estimate include everything, or are there costs I don't know about?
- Who else will be sending me a bill?
- What will the long-term costs be after the patient gets discharged from the hospital?
- Will the patient have to go to a rehabilitation facility, a long-term care facility or sub-acute facility? If so, how much will that cost and who will pay for it?

Insurance coverage:

- Does the insurance company cover the proposed test, treatment or surgery? (Any time a person goes to get medical care, call right away to make sure the insurance company will approve and pay for the visit.)

- What will the insurance company pay for? (When you call the insurance company, make sure you write down whom you talked to, what was said, and what time you called. Ask the person to send you the information in writing.)
- What percentage of the bill is the patient's responsibility?
- Do I need to call the insurance company to get a pre-authorization for the test, treatment or surgery?
- If the insurance company says it will not pay, can I appeal the decision?
- What will happen if the patient has the treatment but I didn't get a pre-authorization from the insurance company?

Financial distress:

- Is it cheaper to go somewhere else for the test, treatment or surgery?
- If the patient doesn't have any insurance, are there any programs that he or she may be eligible for that can help cover the costs?
- Have I talked to the billing department to see what other options are available? (It is better to talk to the billing department right away, because they will be more willing to help you before you get into financial trouble. You may need to ask for the supervisor of the billing department to get the help you need.)
- Does the patient need to apply for Medicaid or MediCal because he or she is out of money?
- What will happen if the patient can't pay the bills?
- How will all of these costs affect the patient's family?
- Is the patient going to need to declare bankruptcy?

Religious or Spiritual Questions

The following questions can be downloaded from my website, TheCaregiversPath.com.

The patient's religious beliefs:

- What is the patient's faith or belief system? (It may be a traditional religion, a personal spiritual connection or no religion.)

- Is the patient actively practicing his or her religion or spirituality?

- Are the doctors aware of the patient's beliefs? If not, what do I need to tell the doctors?

- Does the patient's belief system play a role in his or her other life decisions?

Religion and healthcare:

- Does the patient's belief system play a role in his or her healthcare decisions?

- What does the religion say about the obligation to keep fighting?

- Does the patient's religion say what can and cannot be chosen when it comes to healthcare decisions?

- Does the patient's religion have rules about how the body can be treated?

- Are there certain fasting or food restrictions in the religion?

- Do I need to ask questions about what services may or may not be provided at a religiously affiliated hospital or clinic?

Religious community:

- Can the religious community provide comfort and support for the patient?

- Do I need to call in the patient's religious leader to help make these decisions?

Religion and death and dying:

- What gives the patient's life meaning or purpose?

- What does the patient's religion say about death and dying?

- Does the patient's religion have certain rituals or prayers that are part of the healing or dying process?

- Before the patient dies, should certain things be done in preparation, either spiritually or physically?

- After the patient dies, should certain things be done to prepare and respect the body?

- Is there a hospital chaplain that I can turn to for help?

No religious beliefs:

- How can I show this person respect without using religion?

- How can this person be comforted while dying, without using religion?

- What values and personal beliefs of the patient can guide me when making these decisions?

Religious beliefs of the decision maker:

- When I am making decisions for the patient, how does my religion affect my decision making?

- Am I remembering to respect the beliefs of the patient and to not impose my own religious beliefs? (It is your responsibility to make sure that others involved in the person's care are not imposing their own religious beliefs on the decision making process.)

Cultural Questions

The following questions can be downloaded from my website, TheCaregiversPath.com.

The culture of the patient:

- How much does the patient follow the rules of his or her culture?

- What would the patient say about his or her cultural values and how they would apply in this situation?

- What is the patient's view of the illness in the context of his or her life?

- How would a doctor from the patient's culture handle this situation?

- How would a doctor from the patient's country handle this situation?

- Are there fears, concerns or misperceptions about the proposed treatments because of cultural beliefs?

- Does the patient want to be told the truth about the illness or would the person rather not know?

Choosing the decision maker:

- What does the culture say about who should be the decision maker?
- Should the decision maker be one person or a group of people?

Family involvement:

- What does the patient or the family say would help in this situation?
- Are there community resources available to help the patient when he or she is discharged?

Alternative medicine and healers:

- Is the patient going to a healer, herbalist, spiritual healer or other person for help?
- Do you need to call in a healer or someone to pray?
- Does the patient trust Western medicine?
- Does the patient want to receive the medicines or alternative medications that are used in the patient's country or culture?
- Is the patient taking alternative medications?
- Do I need to tell the doctor the truth about the alternative medications or treatments the patient is receiving outside the doctor's care? (I would recommend telling the truth so your doctor can keep your loved one safe from any side effects of combining what your loved one is taking and what the doctor is prescribing.)

Culture and healthcare:

- Are there certain things the patient can do or not do to get better because of the rules in the culture?
- Are there certain things the patient can eat or not eat to get better?
- Does the patient typically show pain, or does this individual prefer to be brave and accept suffering?
- Are there gender restrictions on who can take care of or touch the patient? If so, what would be okay?
- How would this person want to be shown respect?

Language barriers:

- Does this person speak the same language as the healthcare team, or should a trained medical interpreter be used?
- Are the forms and written information available in the patient's language?
- Can the patient read the forms and the written information about the disease and treatment options?

> I would recommend that a trained medical interpreter always be used when talking to a healthcare professional. Even though it might be easier to use a family member to translate, the family member may not know how to interpret the medical terms that the doctor is using and may end up putting the patient at risk.

Culture and death and dying:

- Are there cultural healing or dying rituals that need to be performed?
- After the person's death, are there rituals that need to be performed or are there certain ways that the body needs to be treated?

The decision maker's cultural beliefs:

- When I am making decisions for the patient, how does my culture affect my decision making?

- Am I remembering to use the culture of the patient and to not impose my own cultural beliefs?

- What else do I need to understand about this person's culture so that I can make good decisions?

When I was making each decision for my dad, I ended up using the same five to ten questions over and over again. I chose the questions that were absolutely necessary. I also was able to ignore some of the questions because they didn't apply to him. And, I didn't need to ask some of them—the answers were obvious because I knew my dad so well. I would encourage you to go through all of the questions the first few times you are making a new decision. Then pick out the questions that will always apply for your loved one. Since my dad was an accountant, I had to make sure I was taking good care of him and his money; asking good financial questions was important. Pick the ones that work for your loved one, but don't forget to occasionally review the other questions and categories. These alternate questions may hold the key to making a good decision. Or if you are struggling because the decision is very difficult, take the time to read through these questions once again. You may find an answer hidden among these lists.

The next set of questions regarding quality of life may become your favorites. I know a few of them are on my list of favorites.

12

Quality of Life and Personal Values

In my work as a bioethics consultant, it doesn't surprise me when one patient says, "I want to take the chance and have another surgery," while another person in the same situation would say, "Absolutely no more surgeries for me." When I start a bioethics consult, I can't begin to guess what a person will say. I have to ask questions to find out what this particular individual thinks is the "right" thing to do. It may be similar to what I think would be right, or it may be completely opposite from what I would do. But it is not my body and it is not my decision. All I can do is to make sure the individual has received plenty of information and has had all of his or her questions answered. It is not for me to say what I think is important; instead I have to discover what is important to the person who is going to receive the treatment. The final decision will be based on the patient's quality-of-life goals.

In this section we will be talking about how to respect what would be meaningful to your loved one and how to discover this individual's quality-of-life goals. Let's begin by taking a look at the difference between a medical goal and a quality-of-life goal.

Medical Goals versus Quality-of-Life Goals

When it comes to making quality-of-life decisions, we have to keep in mind that quality-of-life goals are very different from medical goals. A quality-of-life goal answers the questions "What kind of life does the patient want after he or she is discharged from the hospital?" "What would this individual consider to be a meaningful life?" and "How would this particular person define a valuable existence?" These are the questions that tell us who this person is, what makes this individual unique and what this person's life goals might be. The doctor should try to achieve both the medical goals and the life goals for the patient.

The medical goal answers these types of questions as follows: "The goal of this treatment is to achieve this specific health or medical outcome." "This medicine will make the pain stop." "The surgery will remove the tumor." "The chemotherapy will or will not be able to cure the cancer." Doctors sometimes get caught up in the details of the medical treatment plan and forget to ask questions about the long-term life goals of the patient. They are creating the treatment plan before they know what the patient's personal life goal is in this particular situation. They are doing things in the wrong order. The medical treatment goals should be decided after the doctor understands the quality-of-life goals for this person. Otherwise, the wrong plan might be created. Here are some questions you can use to help you make quality-of-life decisions.

Quality-of-Life Questions

The following questions can be downloaded from my website, TheCaregiversPath.com.

Changes in quality of life:

- Based on the patient's quality of life before this hospitalization or treatment, how has the patient's quality of life changed?
- Is this change in quality of life something that the patient would be willing to live with?
- What would the patient say is an acceptable level of "better"?
- If I don't know, can I find out more about the patient?
- Will the patient be able to return to the same caregivers, friends and family?
- Will the patient be able to return to the same environment?
- If not, how can we help the patient adjust to a new environment?

- Will the patient be able to enjoy his or her meals as before?

- Will the patient be able to enjoy the same activities as before?

If the patient could communicate in the past:

- What would this individual consider to be a meaningful life?

- What kind of life would the patient want after being discharged from the hospital?

- What would the patient say if he or she could talk right now?

- What did the patient say to others in the past about the type of situation he or she is facing?

- What would the patient say is important to consider?

- What would I want, and how is that different from what the patient would want?

The quality-of-life goal and the medical goal:

- Now that we know the quality-of-life goal, can it be achieved medically?

- Is a time-limited trial appropriate to see if the quality-of-life goal and the medical goal can be reached?

- If the quality-of-life goal is not achievable, what level of recovery is possible?

After you figure out the quality-of-life goal, then you and the doctor can work together to determine if the goal is attainable. While it may be hard to accept, your loved one may have a quality-of-life goal that can't be reached. If so, you will have to do your best to discover what else is possible. One question I use is "What would the patient say is an acceptable level of 'better'?" Then you will know what kind of life the person would be willing to put up with and make decisions accordingly. In some situations, the doctor may not agree with what the patient would think is valuable. If you get into a values conflict with the doctor, then you can ask for help from the bioethics committee at the hospital or long-term care facility. Don't wait until the conflict gets worse; ask for help right away.

How Quality-of-Life Goals Can Affect Decisions

Now, let me give you some examples of how much the quality-of-life goal can affect the medical treatment plan.

There are four women in the hospital: Gloria, Maria, Florence and Leena. They have all had massive strokes and unfortunately, they are not going to be able to go back to their regular lives. All four will have to live in sub-acute nursing facilities, will be on ventilators and will not be able to recognize or communicate with their loved ones. (A sub-acute facility has the ability to take care of patients on ventilators.) The doctor for these patients, Dr. Sanchez, can begin to make decisions about what needs to be done for them medically. On the surface, these decisions might look very similar for each of these ladies, but Dr. Sanchez is a smart doctor and realizes that he needs to know more about each woman's quality-of-life goals before he can create a good, individualized medical plan for each of them. He doesn't assume that just because they have had similar strokes that they all want the same things in life.

Gloria's Story

Dr. Sanchez asks Gloria's decision maker, "If Gloria could wake up and tell us what to do, what would she say? What would Gloria say about what makes her life worth living? Would she want to live in a nursing facility on a ventilator and be unable to recognize or communicate with her loved ones?" Her decision maker says, "Gloria wouldn't want to live like this. She was a vibrant, active person and she always said she wouldn't want to live if she couldn't still do the things she loved. Gloria even wrote down that she wouldn't want to be kept alive on machines if she couldn't think anymore."

> Not all decision makers are lucky enough to have had a conversation with their loved one about quality-of-life goals. Sometimes we have to figure out what the patient would want based on other life choices. This is when the decision maker would be using the Substituted Judgment framework and asking the questions on pages 29-30.

Now Dr. Sanchez knows that even though he could put Gloria in a nursing facility, it isn't what Gloria would want. He will need to talk to Gloria's loved ones about withdrawing her from the ventilator and helping her to have a peaceful and dignified death. Now, you might be saying, "I can't believe Gloria would want that. How could she choose to die?" Or perhaps you are saying to yourself, "That is exactly what I would want. I would want to be allowed to die if I were going to be living in that kind of condition." Whatever you are thinking, you are not wrong. That is your opinion, and you should write down what you would want so your future decision maker will know what to do. But this is Gloria's life, and her decision maker is making the right choice to honor Gloria's wishes.

You can begin to see why it is important for the doctor and the loved ones to talk about more than what medicine can do. The medical treatment plan has to fit the patient's life goal, and we all have different life goals.

Maria's Story

Later that day, Dr. Sanchez meets with Maria's family and asks the decision maker, "If Maria could wake up and tell us what to do, what would she say? What would Maria say about what makes her life worth living? Would she want to live in a nursing facility on a ventilator and be unable to recognize or communicate with her loved ones?" Maria's decision maker then says, "Maria is a profoundly religious person and she would say that all life is precious. Maria would still want all of her family to visit her, even if she couldn't recognize them. She would say that being alive in any condition, even a bad condition, is important to her. She wouldn't want us to give up." Now Dr. Sanchez can create the right medical treatment plan for Maria: She can be discharged to the sub-acute nursing facility and can live with a ventilator breathing for her. The treatment plan will fit Maria's quality-of-life goal—her voice has been heard and respected.

Florence's Story

The following day, Dr. Sanchez talks with Florence's loved ones: "If Florence could wake up and tell us what to do, what would she say? What would Florence say about what makes her life worth living? Would she want to live in a nursing facility on a ventilator and be unable to recognize or communicate with her loved ones?" Her daughter says, "Florence never told us what she would want. She would never talk about these issues, even though we tried to talk to her about it." This is when it gets more difficult for the doctor and Florence's decision maker. Without having enough information, the decision maker is going to have to guess what the patient might have wanted. I would recommend going through the questions in the Substituted Judgment section as well as the questions in chapter 11. Florence's decision maker will have to do the best she can to apply what she knows about Florence to the situation. What kind of person was Florence before this happened? What did Florence value?

Leena's Story

Poor Dr. Sanchez—he has one more family to talk to today. It isn't easy for doctors to have these difficult conversations. They have to have a lot of courage to tell patients and families bad news and to deal with end-of-life conversations. One thing that should help Dr. Sanchez in this situation is that Leena had taken the time to fill out an Advance Directive for Healthcare this year, which listed Leena's son, Phil, as her decision maker. Leena also wrote in her Advance Directive that she wouldn't want to live on a ventilator. When Dr. Sanchez walks in the room, Phil says to the doctor, "You have to keep my mom alive." Dr. Sanchez begins to explain that he has to respect the patient's written wishes in the Advance Directive and that Leena said she wouldn't want to live on a ventilator. But Phil says, "I don't care what she said; you have to keep her alive." Phil doesn't realize that his job as the decision maker is to honor the wishes of his mom. His mom specifically stated she didn't want a ventilator, and he should respect her request.

This doesn't mean that making the decision will be easy for Phil. It takes a lot of courage to honor the wishes of someone when you don't agree with what she wants. But that is the job of the decision maker. To make the best decisions based on the values of the patient. Hopefully, Dr. Sanchez will be able to support Phil during this process and understand his grief, while staying true to Leena's wishes. If Phil doesn't want to make these decisions or is unwilling to respect his mother's wishes, then another person can and should be assigned as Leena's decision maker.

Deciding What Makes a Person's Life Worth Living

We have been talking about quality-of-life goals for people who have the ability to express opinions—although they may not have chosen to do so. But what do we do when the patient hasn't been able to tell us what he would want because the person never had the mental ability to express any preferences? We have to use the Best Interest Standard and evaluate the quality of the patient's life by the patient's standards.

Let me explain. In each state, there are nonprofit organizations that serve those individuals who become mentally disabled early in life. These organizations not only help with medical decisions but also help to create a viable life plan for these individuals. They are advocates for the disabled, and they take their jobs seriously. In California, these groups are called Regional Centers, and they have representatives that work with hospitals to ensure that the right decisions are being made.

I was once involved in a case in which a fifty-seven-year-old developmentally disabled man was dying, and the doctors and his conservator were in conflict over the right thing to do. The Regional Center representative was called in to participate in the discussion. The representative made it very clear that his client was entitled to good medical care, including everything that would be offered to other patients. We all agreed, but then we struggled to figure out what would be a good quality-of-life goal for this person. This man's developmental age had never progressed past the age of three, so he hadn't been able to express any values beyond his favorite food.

Many questions were asked at this meeting, including whether or not artificial nutrition should be given through a feeding tube inserted in his stomach while he was dying. Another question was whether or not he could return to the same group home he had been living in, since the home might not be qualified to take care of his medical needs. The representative gave us some insight into this dilemma.

The representative explained that the goal was not to bring the disabled person back to an existence that we would want, but to an existence that the disabled person would want. When an individual has a limited ability to interact with the world, we have to try to see the world as he or she experiences it. The representative explained that for a person with limited mental abilities, it would be meaningful to be able to return to the same familiar environment with familiar smells, familiar noises, familiar caregivers and a familiar schedule. The disabled need continuity throughout their lives and especially when dying. Because of our patient's limited capacity, it would be more difficult for him to adjust to new surroundings. It would be like taking a young child out of his family's home and making the child live with a new family. That would be traumatic.

Here are some of the questions the representative said we should be asking in this case:

- Is he able to return to the same caregivers and friends?
- Is he able to return to the same environment?
- Will he be able to adjust to a new environment?
- Is he able to enjoy his meals as he could before?

We first tackled the feeding tube issue. The representative, who knew this person well, said that for this patient, the difference between enjoying his meals and getting his food through a tube represented a substantial loss for him. One of the few pleasures this man had was his ability to taste food. He loved to eat. Losing this ability would severely decrease the quality of his life—by his own standards. If this same patient had already been on a feeding tube, then continuing the feeding tube would not be a difficult choice to make because it wouldn't change his quality of life.

This already difficult decision was further complicated by the fact that this man was days away from dying, and most people naturally stop eating when they are close to death. While considering this issue, we had to keep in mind our obligation to the disabled to make sure they are fed. We also had to think about the risks involved with the procedure to insert the feeding tube. The other concern that weighed heavily on our scale as we balanced the benefits and the burdens was that if he had the feeding tube put in, he couldn't go back to his group home. He would have to go somewhere new for the last days of his life.

This situation was complex and there was no easy answer. As the group considered all of these issues and other relevant information, the decision was made to not insert the feeding tube. I am not saying this is the right decision in all situations, but this decision was in the best interest of this particular man at that time. This is what makes ethical medical decision making complicated. Once you have the tools, you still have to think about the details of the situation and how the different options will play out.

We then tackled the question of whether this man should return to the group home or stay in the hospital. You and I might not want to live in a group home because we expect a different quality of life. But for this patient, that was his home. He had lived there for years and the people there were his family. It would have been a tremendous loss for him to be away from his family of caregivers. Being able to return to the group home where he lived was a worthwhile goal for him, even if he only had a few days to live. The plan was to have hospice support him when he returned home and to help him have a good death.

This was a powerful experience for me because it reminded me not only to use the values of the patient, but also to truly step inside this person's existence to feel what brings this individual happiness, comfort and a meaningful life. As we have discussed, think about it from the specific person's perspective. When you begin to make quality-of-life decisions for your loved one, please remember to think about what would be valuable to your loved one, not to you.

With each situation we face, we need to adjust our view of what constitutes a good life. Just because we might not want to live like another person doesn't mean that this individual is not experiencing a good life. Keep in mind that we are making decisions for a unique individual, not a generic disabled person. We need to make these decisions very carefully, as our loved ones will experience the consequences of *our* decisions. Whether our decision is an easy medical decision or an end-of-life decision, we need to protect our loved one and help give voice to his other needs. In the next section, we are going to focus on making the most difficult decisions, the end-of-life decisions.

THE END OF LIFE

13

Making the Most Difficult Decisions at the End of Life

I know this may be a difficult section for many people to read, but if you have made it this far, then you probably have the courage to keep going. I hope you have a long time with your loved one and that all you need this book for is to help with the decision making process. But if you want to be more prepared, you may want to read this last section now so that when the time comes, you will know what to expect and won't be making decisions in a crisis. You will already know what needs to be done.

The other reason I hope you will read this section early on is that you will need to make sure that the doctor understands the values and quality-of-life goals of your loved one. As we have already discussed, medicine is rushed and people forget to stop and ask the meaningful questions. You need to make sure that the right questions are being asked and that the doctors are hearing your loved one's answers. This will be your last chance to honor and to give voice to his or her needs. You have profound work to do. I think that as you begin to read this section, you will find it less scary to think about than you thought it would be. I will try to help you feel safe as we journey through the process of dying.

What Does Your Loved One Deserve?

Your loved one deserves a good death. We all do. What makes a good death? It is different for every person. I believe that one of the best options for a peaceful and dignified death is what you get when you are on hospice. But you may have something else in mind for how you would like to die. In one nursing bioethics class I was teaching, I asked the nurses, "How do you want to die?" After they got over the shock of being asked such a serious question, they came up with the most amazing answers. Here is what they told me.

- "I want to die in a sacred place. It doesn't have to be a religious place, but a place where I can feel a sense of peace and serenity while being surrounded by my loved ones."

- "I want to die at home. I don't want to be hooked up to machines in the hospital. And I definitely don't want to be in pain."

- "I want to die alone. I don't think I could bear to have my loved ones in the room when it is my time to go. I don't think I would be able to let go."
- "I want my husband and my children surrounding me, singing hymns."
- "I want to die quickly. I would hate to linger."
- "I want to have enough time to say my goodbyes. I would like my death to take a week so everybody I love could come by to see me."

Their answers were unique and special to them. There is no one right answer to how to have a good death. It is a personal and private decision. But be careful not to keep it too private. If nobody knows what you want, you probably won't get it. I would encourage you to start talking about it now.

As your loved one's decision maker, you are in charge of making sure that the person with diminished capacity gets the best death possible. I know that sounds strange. But don't you fight to get good medical care? Haven't you been working hard to make sure he or she has the best life care that is possible? Then why wouldn't you fight just as hard to get the person what he or she needs when dying? Since this individual probably won't be able to tell you what that will be, it is up to you to think in advance about what this person would want. Or if your loved

> Think about how difficult it is for you to make these important decisions for your loved one. Wouldn't you want to make it easier for the people who care about you? The gift of talking about your wishes and what would make your dying profound is the gift we give to each other. You have to be brave enough to bring it up.

one is in the early stages of the disease, talk to him now, while he can still share his thoughts with you.

- What would this individual tell you if he or she could?
- Where would the person want to die?
- Whom would your loved one want to be with?
- What would he or she want you to do as death approaches?
- What would bring peace and comfort during the dying process?
- What does your loved one still need to accomplish to have peace?

You have important decisions to make. Let me give you some more information about your different options to make this a little easier.

Making Decisions about CPR and DNR

CPR or cardiopulmonary resuscitation used to be very simple to understand. *Cardio* stands for heart, *pulmonary* stands for lungs and *resuscitation* means to revive from death. When a patient died, someone would push on the person's chest to try to restart the heart while giving mouth-to-mouth resuscitation to help the person breathe. Over time, CPR has become more complex as healthcare professionals have discovered different and advanced ways to try to bring the person back to life. The patient may be given medications, her heart may be electrically shocked with paddles placed on the chest, and she may be placed on a ventilator to help her breathe. And every year, the researchers find new ways to adapt the CPR process to try to save more lives. What seemed like an easy question, "Does the person want CPR?" has turned into a more complicated decision.

| CPR: Cardiopulmonary resuscitation |
| DNR: Do not resuscitate |
| DNAR: Do not attempt resuscitation |
| AND: Allow natural death |

The doctor may at some point ask you, "Should the patient be made a DNR?" DNR means *do not resuscitate* or do not do CPR. It is interesting to me that we have three ways to say do *not* do CPR: DNR, DNAR and AND. Yet the differences are very important. Do not *attempt* resuscitation (DNAR) more appropriately describes the situation. Just because you attempt CPR doesn't mean it will work. The doctor is being truthful when she asks you, "Should we *attempt* CPR." She is not making any false promises that CPR will work. The newest term, AND (or *allow natural death*), is a more gentle way of saying *do not resuscitate*. Instead of telling you what won't be done for your loved one, the doctor is offering to allow your loved one a peaceful, natural death and will not attempt resuscitation.

This will be a difficult decision for you to make, and I want you to be prepared. It should be handled just like the other medical decisions you have had to make. Using the tools from the earlier sections, you should be able to determine whether the person should be involved in the decision making or not. If you have the patient's Advance Directive, what does it say? If you are using Substituted Judgment, then you should consider what the person would say if she could wake up and understand what was going on. If you are using the Best Interest Standard, then you have to ask yourself what a generic person would want in this situation.

But before you can fully answer this question, you will want to find out what risks are involved and what the chances are that CPR will work on your loved one. I've asked many groups of healthcare professionals, "How many of you would like to die by CPR?" No one ever, ever raises a hand. What is it that they know that they're not telling us? They know that the chance of CPR working is minimal, sometimes even 0 percent.

Doctors rarely tell you that what you see on television is wrong, so I will have to be the bearer of bad news. On shows like *ER*, CPR brings the patient back to life about 75 percent of the time (Diem, Lantos and Tulsky 1996), when in real life it only works, at best, 17 percent of the time (Peberdy, et al. 2003). In some situations, the chance of success is zero. The shows also mislead you by letting you think a person will be healthy enough to go home about 67 percent of the time (Diem, Lantos and Tulsky 1996). In reality, if CPR is able to bring the patient back to life, the chance of this person going home with good brain function is about 7 percent (Kaldjian, et al. 2009). Some patients may survive CPR but are never able to leave the hospital. Others may remain hooked up to ventilators for the rest of their lives. The success rate will depend on the health of the patient, the patient's age, how quickly the CPR was begun and other medical factors. These results and statistics are for those who are healthy and need CPR. Unfortunately, there are times when CPR won't work no matter how much you want it to.

William J. Ehlenbach, MD, lead author of a study of CPR in the elderly, published in the *New England Journal of Medicine* in 2009, explains, "CPR has the highest likelihood of success when the heart is the reason, as in an ongoing heart attack or a heart rhythm disturbance. If you're otherwise doing well, CPR will often be successful. But, if you're in the ICU [intensive care unit] with a serious infection and multiple organ failure, it's unlikely that CPR will save you" (quote from Gordon 2009; study published by Ehlenbach et al. 2009).

To make the decision about CPR, you will need to ask the doctor to give you more information about the chance of CPR working for your loved one's specific condition and what the risks of CPR would be (what negative situations could result from CPR). The doctor may have to look up the recent statistics for your loved one's condition, or you could do the research yourself. I know that for many patients and families, it is difficult to accept that CPR doesn't work 75 percent of the time as it does on television, and that the real chances for success are 0 to 17 percent. When you have clear, factual information, you will be able to make a more informed decision.

I often find that doctors don't really describe what can happen when CPR is performed. Your loved one may be brought back to life but in a worse condition than before, both mentally and physically. When the healthcare team is pushing on the person's chest, there is a chance of broken ribs or a collapsed lung. The longer the patient isn't able to breathe, the greater the chance for brain damage. There may also be damage to the windpipe if the person is placed on a ventilator. For many people, CPR just prolongs the dying process.

A new form that is being used by physicians is called a POLST form. POLST stands for Physician Orders for Life-Sustaining Treatments. This is a doctor's order form that documents the patient's wishes, not only about CPR but for other end-of-life choices as well. When you have a POLST form, your wishes will be respected whether you are in the hospital, the ambulance, a long-term care facility or your home. In your state, this form may have a slightly different name, such as MOLST, or Medical Orders for Life-Sustaining Treatments. The POLST form may or may not be available where you live. You can ask your doctor about it.

Another concern is that the person might not have the opportunity for a peaceful and profound death experience. When you picture the last minutes of your loved one's life, do you see strangers straddling the patient on a bed, pushing on the patient's chest, while the family waits outside the door? Or do you see a time with family and friends gathered around the bedside, with words of love being expressed, music being played or prayers being said?

I am not saying that you shouldn't choose to attempt CPR; I just want to make sure you have the facts about the chances of it working and about what kind of condition your loved one might be in afterward. Just like making other medical decisions, you should balance the benefits and the burdens or risks so that you can make a good decision.

If I Say, "No CPR," Does That Mean Everything Stops?

Sometimes doctors confuse the decision about CPR with decisions about all of the other treatment options. But no, the decision about CPR is just one part of the treatment plan. A patient may want chemotherapy, surgery, radiation therapy or other kinds of aggressive treatments and still may want to be a DNR. Or the person may not want other medical treatments but still want to receive CPR. These are all separate decisions and any combination is possible. One choice shouldn't limit the other options. Choose some, choose all or choose none. It is up to you to make the decisions that your loved one would want you to make. The only thing you can't choose is a treatment that is not a valid medical option. You cannot make the doctor give your loved one ineffective or non-beneficial treatments. And sometimes, CPR falls into that category because it is a non-beneficial treatment that simply won't work.

So, when the doctor says, "Would your loved one want CPR?" give the doctor your answer and then tell the doctor about where and how this person would want to die. Help the doctor have a more meaningful conversation. A few doctors won't ask you the CPR question because they want to avoid the topic, so you may have to begin the conversation. You're going to have to teach some doctors to be brave and to be willing to talk with you about these important issues. You're going to have to ask for clear answers and for the support you need. And if the doctor won't talk to you and your loved one, find a doctor who will. And if after talking with the doctor, you realize he won't respect or support your loved one's wishes, find a doctor who will.

When Your Loved One Gets CPR Against Her Will

Dear Viki,

I just got the call that my mother-in-law, who is in end-stage Alzheimer's, was resuscitated (got CPR) twice even though she had a DNR order in place. Instead of being allowed to die, she is now in the ICU receiving care she doesn't want. What just happened? What do I do next?

My answer:

Even though this isn't supposed to ever happen, occasionally it does. A DNR, or a do not resuscitate, order should be followed, but sometimes people are in a hurry or they don't check the chart or they don't agree with the order. Then a person, like your mother-in-law, is brought back to life against her will. This is a terrible thing for the patient and family to go through. The person's wishes are not being respected and she doesn't get to die a natural death.

Here is the legal truth about this situation. If the healthcare professionals knew that there was a DNR in place, then what they did to your mother-in-law is called *assault and battery*. The healthcare professionals involved can be arrested and criminally charged. And I need to let any healthcare professionals who might be reading this know that your malpractice insurance won't cover this because it is a criminal offense. If the healthcare team didn't know that she wanted to be a DNR, then you need to make sure the doctor writes the DNR order immediately so that it won't happen again.

What can you do now that it has happened? The best thing to do is to talk to the nursing supervisor and find out if the staff realizes they made a mistake. (Don't be hostile or aggressive, as these caregivers are still taking care of your mother-in-law.) Be polite and make sure that there really is a DNR order written on the chart and that it will be respected in the future. Sometimes we think these instructions have been written, but the doctor hasn't gotten around to it—or perhaps the doctor won't write it because of moral opposition to the DNR order. Doctors are allowed to live by their morals and to refuse to participate in acts that go against their values. But they are still obligated to let you know about valid medical options and then let the patient/decision maker decide. If the doctor doesn't want to do this, then the doctor should help you find a doctor who is willing to talk to the patient and you about the appropriate options that are available. If the doctor won't write the DNR and won't talk to you or the patient about it, then fire that doctor and get another doctor to write it.

The first people you should ask for help are the nursing supervisor or the social worker. They will know whom to call and will help advocate for the patient. If you continue to have problems, you can always call the hospital's bioethics committee for help. Just call the hospital operator and ask for the bioethics committee, and you will be connected to the right person. When there is a serious problem in a hospital after hours, you can call the hospital operator, who will notify the hospital administrator who is on call that night. Help is available, but you have to keep asking until you get to the right person who can resolve the issue.

A follow-up note: I spoke with the daughter-in-law directly and found out that although the family thought the patient had a DNR, she really only had an Advance Directive that said do not resuscitate. Those wishes were not transferred onto the hospital chart. You need to be careful: Even though the patient may have refused a certain treatment in the Advance Directive, it won't take effect until someone on the healthcare team is made aware and it is written in the patient's chart. Without doctor's orders written in the patient's chart, the patient's wishes won't be followed. In this situation, it was not a lack of respect for the person, just a lack of communication. The lesson to learn here is to make sure you go over your loved one's Advance Directive and other healthcare wishes with the doctor when you arrive at the hospital.

When Your Loved One Said to Do Everything, but Everything Isn't Possible

Dear Viki,

My father said he wanted everything done, but I can't bear to watch his suffering. It seems like he keeps getting these terrible treatments but nothing works. The doctor keeps asking me if I think it is time to put him on hospice but I promised my dad that I would make sure the doctor didn't give up on him. My dad is the type of person who would never give in or give up. I feel like I am supposed to do what he says, but isn't there ever a time when I should just say, "Enough"?

My answer:

I am so sorry you are in this terrible position. It must be difficult to balance doing what you think is the right thing for your dad with trying to respect his wishes. The first thing I would suggest is to make sure you get better pain management for your dad. He shouldn't be suffering while he fights his disease. Ask for a referral to a palliative care doctor. This type of doctor can help you with the healing of your dad's suffering and will help get his symptoms under control.

Secondly, what you are experiencing is moral distress—you are doing the right thing but it feels so wrong. For some people, there is tremendous value in fighting to the end. Not giving up is more important than the hardships that are faced along the way. But this can put a tremendous burden on the person having to make these decisions and witness the results. The other people who suffer greatly are the healthcare professionals who have to participate by inflicting care that they don't think is helping the patient anymore.

It is so painful when our loved one asks us to advocate for things we don't agree with. The thing you have to realize is that this is your dad's life and health. People have the right to make bad decisions. You have to be brave enough to do right by your dad and respect his bad decision.

The rest of the answer to your question:

Here are your obligations. Since your dad told you that he wanted to fight to the end, that is what you should try to do. If there are more treatments that the doctor can try, then you should have the doctor keep trying to find what will work to cure your dad. If the treatments are only causing suffering and are not helping your dad, then you are not obligated to continue with the plan. You are supposed to fight for the medical options that will actually benefit your dad. Talk to the doctor and ask if there is something else that should be tried. If there is nothing else that the doctor can offer, that is when you can say, "Enough." Then you will need to advocate for the best end-of-life care you can. When the time comes, you can fight for a pain-free and peaceful death. Don't think of this as giving up; think of it as fighting for a different goal when the time comes.

What Is the Difference Between Palliative Care, Comfort Care and Hospice Care?

Dear Viki,

My wife's doctor told me it is time for her to have comfort care, and they sent in a palliative care doctor. I'm kind of confused because I don't understand the difference between hospice care, palliative care and comfort care. Is there a difference between these, and if not, why do each of the doctors say different things when they talk to me? What is the doctor trying to tell me about my wife?

My answer:

I think sometimes even doctors and nurses get confused by these different words to describe pain management and end-of-life care. The words do mean different things, but many times they are used to describe the same thing—the support your loved one will get during the process of dying. In practice, doctors may be saying the same things even though they are using different terms. Let me try to explain.

Let's start with *palliative care*. This is the most misunderstood term because it describes two things: pain and symptom management when you're healthy, and the support you receive during the dying process. Palliative care is the global term used to describe all of the care that is related to relieving suffering. To palliate means to relieve or lessen without curing, to mitigate or to alleviate. So your wife might go to a palliative care specialist, even though she is not dying, to help her get her pain under control or to alleviate her physical symptoms. In that situation, the doctor would be there to give your wife good pain management. At another time, your wife might be sent to palliative care to help her with the symptoms of dying. It frustrates palliative care specialists when people think that all they do is take care of the dying. This isn't true. They take care of the suffering of all patients, the living and the dying.

By comparison, *hospice care* is for people in the process of dying. A patient can get palliative care without dying, but you can't get hospice care without being a dying patient. (The exception is for children who can sometimes be receiving medical treatments and be on hospice at the same time.) There are also different kinds of hospices, both volunteer hospices and medical hospices. I volunteer at a volunteer hospice, and we provide respite care and support for the patient and family. We are like good friends who stop by to help out.

A medical hospice will provide visits from nurses, doctors, nursing aides, social workers, volunteers and chaplains. The patient will also be provided medications for symptom management, medical equipment, oxygen, a hospital bed, etc. Everything is provided at no cost to the patient or family.

Hospice care can also be found in different locations. It doesn't always happen in the patient's home. It can also be found in outpatient hospices, in inpatient designated beds in hospitals, in skilled nursing facilities, in board and care facilities, in group homes or in assisted living facilities. Your location shouldn't determine your eligibility for hospice, although there are a few facilities that are not accredited to treat hospice patients.

Now let's talk about *comfort care*. This is a term that is most often used inside of a hospital. Your wife's doctor came in and he talked to you about putting your wife on comfort care. Here is what the doctor is trying to say. He is saying that at this point he has nothing else to offer that could cure your loved one's disease. But what he can offer is to keep her comfortable and to help her have a good death. When he says this, he may not mean that your wife is dying immediately, but that the aggressive treatments are no longer working. He is not abandoning her, but he is changing the focus from curing to caring.

Now, maybe you're saying to yourself, isn't the relief of suffering palliative care? Isn't comfort care palliative care? This is where it gets confusing again. Remember that palliative care is used both when someone is fighting the disease and when someone is in the dying process. In reality, patients should be getting palliative care throughout their medical treatment experience. But sometimes palliative care is brought in very late and only as part of the comfort care (dying) plan. So whether it is time for comfort care or if there are still medical treatment options that will be tried, you will want to speak up and ask for good palliative support. Make sure you advocate for good pain and symptom management both while your loved one is healing and later on when she is dying. Doctors now know how to take care of these symptoms, but if your doctor doesn't or won't help, then ask for a referral to someone who can. You are lucky. It sounds like your doctor is doing the right thing by asking the palliative care doctor to see your wife.

So, back to your question: If the doctor in the hospital says comfort care, I am sorry to say he means dying care. If he says palliative care in the hospital, he probably means dying care, but he might just mean suffering care. You will need to ask the physician to explain what the *goal* of palliative care is for your wife.

If a doctor wants to make your wife comfort care in the hospital, that means she can probably go home on hospice or perhaps to a facility that can handle her medical condition with hospice support. If your wife wants to die at home, you need to advocate for her and say, "She would like to go home on hospice." You need to speak up about where and how your loved one would like to die. She is entitled to a good death and when it is your time, so are you.

How Do I Get My Loved One on Hospice?

Dear Viki,

How do I get my significant other into hospice? He has cancer that has spread everywhere, and his pain is not being managed. I have heard about hospice, but I don't know whom to call. What can I do?

My answer:

I am so glad you asked. To get a patient on hospice, a doctor has to make the referral to the local medical hospice. You have to ask the doctor, and it could be any of his doctors, to call the hospice and set it up. Some doctors are not willing to put a patient on hospice because they don't want to give up trying. So if your loved one's doctor won't put him on hospice, ask another doctor you know to make the call. Or, you can also call your local hospice and ask the medical director of the hospice to help you. An emergency room doctor can also put someone on hospice.

After the doctor makes the referral, a hospice representative will call you later that day or the next morning. A social worker and a nurse will both be coming out to see your significant other within twenty-four hours. They will evaluate what the patient needs and what your family may need. If he qualifies for hospice, you will start receiving visits from other hospice staff and deliveries of medical supplies such as a hospital bed, oxygen or a bedside commode. You will also be receiving medications to take care of his pain and other symptoms. The hospice team does not provide full-time care, however.

The good news is that none of this will cost you anything. The services will be covered as an insurance benefit through Medicare, Medicaid, MediCal or your private insurance. You will receive a statement from your insurance, but it won't be a bill. If you don't have insurance, there are hospices that take care of patients without insurance or the money to pay. The rules and regulations about hospice services, qualifications and costs change every year. You may want to check with your local hospice for more up-to-date information when the time comes.

A visiting nurse will teach you about the new medicines, and there is a twenty-four-hour hotline you can call if his symptoms change and you need help. Every patient is different. What your loved one will need may be very different than what my dad needed. The good thing about hospice is that as a patient's health needs change, the hospice team can adapt the plan and continue to provide comfort for your loved one.

It may be overwhelming for the first few days, as so many hospice workers will be coming and going as they make sure the patient is well taken care of. Unfortunately, you do lose some privacy, which takes some time to get used to. Don't worry, though—after a while you will get to know the hospice team and they will become your trusted friends. Most people find hospice to be a huge comfort because they know that their loved one won't be alone and suffering.

If your loved one is not getting the services he needs or you don't think that things are going as they should, make sure you speak up and advocate for him. Just like any other business, occasionally a hospice won't live up to its professional obligations. If you are having trouble getting the appropriate services, you should transfer your loved one to a different hospice.

When the Doctor Won't Put Your Loved One on Hospice

Over and over again, I've sat in rooms with thirty doctors and asked the question, "How many of you refer patients to hospice? How early or late?" Out of the thirty doctors, perhaps five will raise their hand. Of those doctors making the referral to hospice, the referral is made very close to the patient's death. This is terrible. Patients and their loved ones are being denied a wonderful service that doesn't cost them anything.

The following section is written for doctors in particular, but everyone should read it. It outlines the things I teach doctors about referring patients to hospice. Copy this section and give it to your loved one's doctor. You can also download this letter and other helpful documents at TheCaregiversPath.com.

Hospice Information for Doctors

An attending doctor does not have to be certain that it is time for the patient to be placed on hospice to make a referral. The medical director at the hospice, who is also a doctor, will evaluate the person to determine if the patient will meet the criteria for hospice. Don't hesitate to make the referral based on finances. Even a patient without insurance or money can receive the hospice benefits for free. A hospice referral is similar to a referral to any other specialist. The patient's regular doctor can still be the primary doctor, and the patient may return to the doctor's office or hospital for care. But the focus of care is now on comfort, support and symptom management. Aggressive treatments won't be offered anymore.

As the patient's primary doctor, the patient still needs you. Even though you are no longer able to heal the disease, you can heal this person's suffering. You can make sure the patient is getting good pain management and good symptom control, and you can help your patient have a profound and meaningful death. Hospice is a wonderful tool to help your patient on his or her journey toward a good death.

Hospice offers a team of people who help meet the patient's physical, psychological, social and spiritual needs. Hospice provides support for both the patient and the loved ones. Research has found that being on hospice will increase both the quality and quantity of the person's remaining days (Connor et al. 2007). Wouldn't you want to live longer and better, even if your days were numbered? I would, and I would want that for those I care about as well.

The referral to the hospice team can be done at any time. Sooner is better than later. Not only is it better for the patient, it is better for the family. The hospice team is there to heal the suffering of the patient as well as the family. After the death, the family will receive bereavement support for twelve to eighteen months. Your patient brought you this handout for a reason; the patient is telling you that he or she is ready for hospice. Please consider referring your patient to hospice so this person can get the care and support he or she needs.

Communicating with the Dying

There are many layers to communicating with the dying. It depends on who the person is, how he or she is dealing with the process of dying, your relationship with this person and many other factors. You may find that one communication strategy will be appropriate for this individual, but that the other parts won't. You will have to do the best you can in the situation you find yourself in each day.

I didn't know all of this myself until about six years ago, when I became a hospice volunteer. I had aging relatives for whom I was responsible, and I felt helpless when it came to dealing with their deaths. So I went through extensive training and have been learning ever since. I would like to share with you what I have learned. I will first discuss the months before the death, and then I will discuss the last days and hours. Both are profoundly important.

The Journey through the Early Days of Dying

Many times when I meet a new hospice family, the family will share with me that the patient doesn't know that she is dying. Then when I sit with the dying person, she will tell me that her family doesn't know she is dying. How can this be? How can they both not realize that the other person already knows what is going on? The family and the patient both want to avoid talking about the fact that death is approaching. They are trying to protect each other and to avoid making the other person or people cry. But what also ends up happening is that the dying person doesn't get to talk about her fears and concerns, and the family members don't get the opportunity to say what is important to them. This lack of conversation can be lonely and isolating for all the people involved.

People want a safe person to talk to; perhaps you can be that person. If you can, you will be giving the gift of conversation, whether it is with your friend, your loved one or someone you are working with in your professional life.

As a side note, I struggle to find the right conversation path when someone doesn't want to talk. I have to remind myself that this is this person's journey, not mine. I am only there to support and to be present if she needs me. I tell my hospice patients that I would be glad to talk about any fears, concerns or hopes for how their death might go. But I accept it when they say, "No, thank you." Maybe they will be ready another time, or maybe I am not the right person for this discussion and they would prefer to talk to someone else. I don't take it personally. I stay present and meet them where they are emotionally that day. I don't try to push them when they aren't ready. That would be disrespectful.

Keep in mind that everyone is unique. Let the person guide you through the conversation. You may find that on some days the person will have a lot of questions, and on other days he will just want to talk about the game last night.

This list is just a starting place for you to understand what might be on the mind of someone who is dying:

- To know the diagnosis and prognosis, in order to make good medical and life decisions
- To be treated as a person and not just as a body in the bed
- To be at home or wherever the person would prefer
- To talk about any fears of pain, physical decline, increasing dependence, and the loss of dignity and control
- To talk about any spiritual crisis he or she is experiencing
- To have any moods understood, such as anger, sadness, hopelessness, guilt, denial or frustration
- To be able to express his or her grief to those who are willing to listen
- To feel that dying is a natural process and it's okay to let go
- To be able to communicate honestly with family and friends
- To be as pain-free and alert as possible, for as long as possible
- To be in as much control as possible until the end
- To know that the person's family and friends will be okay after he or she is gone

- To be shown respect and compassion by those who are doing the caregiving
- To be able to complete unfinished business
- To be able to ignore the dying process and not complete any unfinished business
- To be given a sense of purpose during the remaining days
- To find meaning in what is being experienced

The Journey through the Final Days of Dying

Not everyone will die in the same way or with the same symptoms. But I would like to tell you about some of the common signs we see with our hospice patients as they move through the last stages of dying. Don't worry if what I describe isn't exactly how it ends up being for your loved one. Everyone dies in his or her own time and own way. And don't worry if some of the things that happen are things I haven't mentioned. This is just an overview of the process. I just want to help you be less afraid and understand that dying is normal. Hopefully, your loved one has the support of a good hospice team and the hospice nurse can answer any other questions you might have.

A few hours before my dad died, a couple of his friends stopped by to say their goodbyes. His friend Mary asked me, "What do you think your dad would be saying right now?" I said, "He would probably say that dying is difficult because we haven't done it before." The reason I told her this was because he used to say the same thing about aging: "Getting older is difficult because we haven't done it before."

How true both of these statements are; anything that is unknown to us can be scary. If we had done it before, we would know that it isn't as bad as we thought it would be. We might realize that there can be profound lessons in aging and in dying. We might be more at peace during the dying process because we would know that our bodies know how to die.

What do I mean by this? The act of dying is sometimes referred to as the labor of death. It is actually rather similar to the labor of birth, though hopefully a lot less painful. Let me explain. When you were about to be born, your mother didn't have to say to her uterus, "Please contract now and begin to push the baby out" or "Cervix, please dilate so the baby can come out." Your mother's body knew what to do and the labor of birth happened naturally. The labor of death is similar to the labor of birth because our bodies know what to do. We don't need to be afraid. We knew how to be born and we know how to die.

Our bodies go through predictable and peaceful changes as death approaches. As we begin to near the end of life, we may begin to sleep more and to become less interested in the world around us. We may not have the strength to do the things we used to do. When we are getting closer to death, maybe during the last few days or hours, our bodies begin to change. We are probably sleeping all the time and are too weak to open our eyes. Our bodies know that it's time to shut down and that we don't need extra food to keep us going. When we are no longer eating or drinking, our electrolytes get out of balance and that affects our brain. (The electrolytes work as a balancing system, keeping all of the chemicals in our body working in balance together. Without the proper balance, our brain and bodily functions are affected.) In our last hours, our skin will get cooler or we may get a fever. Or we may fluctuate between being really hot and being really cold. Our breathing patterns will change back and forth from being very fast to being slow or barely there. There are many other symptoms that we may also experience.

Not only are there physical changes during the last days of life, but caregivers may begin to see unusual interactions. Let me share with you some of the common experiences witnessed by those who do hospice work. The dying may begin to speak of being in the presence of those who have already died. This frightens many families, and some people try to argue with the dying, saying, "You are wrong" or "You are confused." Why do you need to argue? Your loved one is dying! Instead, ask the person questions: "Who do you see? What do you see? Tell me about it." I expected my father to see his mama and papa, whom he missed dearly and adored. But he started talking to the empty space right next to me and kept saying, "Martin." I asked, "Mama?" But he said, "No, Martin." Then it hit me. His best friend in his younger years was Martin. His dearest friend had come to guide him on his journey. Now, some people say it is just the electrolytes affecting the brain and triggering old memories. Others say that it is truly a guide coming to escort the person to the afterlife. I don't know which is true, but I have been privileged to witness this part of the journey.

Another thing that may happen is that the dying will speak of preparing to travel or to change. My dad did this. He kept saying, "The train is late. I have to get on the train." I have seen this many times. Sometimes it is a bus or a plane or another form of transportation, but it is a message that tells us that the time is getting closer. Other people will talk of seeing a place. Again, ask about it. Reassure the person if he or she is confused or frightened. Let your loved one know that he is safe and that what he is seeing is okay.

Some people will know the time of their death or will keep asking what time it is. Or perhaps when you leave and you say, "See you tomorrow," the dying person might say, "No, you won't." Sometimes it is absolutely true and sometimes it is just wishful thinking as the person is getting ready for the journey. The main thing to remember is that the confusion is normal. Your loved one is disconnecting from this world and letting go of what has held him here. The mind is somewhere else now. This is okay. Again, don't argue or judge or discount the experience. Enjoy the ride with the person.

An unusual thing that can happen is that a few days or a few hours before death, the person may have a sudden burst of energy. For some reason, some people who have been sleeping all of the time suddenly wake up and start talking again. This can be very confusing for the family. They believe that a miracle is happening, that the person is going to get better. They don't realize what is really happening—that death is even closer. I have been told that this has also been seen in animals. My friend Amber told me about her beloved horse's last days. He couldn't leave the stall or walk anymore, but the day before he died, he got a sudden burst of energy and went out and played with the other horses in the field for a few hours. The vet had warned her about this phenomenon, so she looked at it as a gift. Her horse had one more bright moment in his life. And then, hours later, he died a good death. So enjoy the moment, if you are lucky enough to get it. If someone comes back to you for a few minutes or hours, remember that it will not last forever. Say anything else you need to say, and be grateful you got the chance.

Near the very end, the person will probably become completely unresponsive. That doesn't mean that he or she can't still hear you or feel your touch. Talk to your loved one as if the person is still with you. Be cautious about talking about things you wouldn't usually discuss when the person was in the room. I have witnessed families saying, "So what does the will say?" or "How much do you think we will get?" in the room with the dying patient. Step outside and have these types of discussions in a more private place.

One of the best ways to communicate with the dying is by touch. Put some lotion on the person's hands or feet, and give the individual a massage. Climb into bed and take your loved one into your arms. Think about how you would comfort children. You would stroke their head, cuddle with them and help them *feel* loved.

As death approaches, tell your loved one that it's okay to go. People will hold on for a long time, waiting to hear these words. They want you to say something like, "I will miss you, but I will be okay. The family will be okay. You taught me what I need to know. We will take care of each other. When it is time, it is okay for you to go." Or any words that will make it safe for the person to let go.

Also, remember that some people need to die alone to protect their loved ones. Over and over again, nurses will tell me of a spouse who sits at the bedside day after day. The spouse never leaves to bathe or to eat. And finally, after days of waiting, the spouse gives in and says, "I am just going to run and get a cup of coffee in the cafeteria." As soon as the spouse leaves, the patient dies. When the spouse comes back, he is devastated that he wasn't there when the time came. I know people who have been shattered by this experience. They didn't know that their loved one was protecting them and didn't want to put them through the possible trauma of witnessing his or her death. It wasn't that the spouse didn't matter; it was that the spouse mattered too much. My dad kept holding on for days and days. Finally I said to him, "I know you need to do this alone. I am going to go now, Dad. I love you and I know you won't be here when I get back. Goodbye." I went outside and twenty minutes later he was gone. I was glad he was able to let go and do it his way. People have to die on their own terms. We can't control the process.

At the opposite end of the spectrum, many patients can't let go until either a certain person or group of people have arrived. My recent hospice patient was like that. I was surprised he was still there when I visited him. He had every physical symptom of impending death, but he was still holding on. I realized his sister was due in about three hours, and then I understood. He held on for his sister's visit and then he died peacefully.

You won't know what your loved one will need until you are in the moment. Whatever happens is okay. You don't have to be perfect; just be present and loving. Try to do whatever you can to give comfort and support. Maybe you could hold your loved one's hand or play his favorite songs. Above all, make sure that the religious or cultural dying rituals that need to be performed are done.

This journey is also about those who will remain after the person is gone. At this time, people should do what is meaningful, both to the dying and to those who are grieving. I tell the families I work with in hospice, "Do what you need to do.

At the end of this, you have to have peace that you were able to say and do those things that were important to you." As the caregiver, you will need comfort and support as you walk this path with your loved one. This includes those who are professional caregivers; you are grieving too. Reach out and ask for the support you need.

I always feel so honored to be a part of a person's final days, whether I get to be present in the early days as the individual is coming to terms with approaching death or during the last moments of life. It is an incredibly intimate experience and one that I have been privileged to be a part of many times. I hope you can find the beauty and profound nature of the experience as well.

Did I Matter?

One of the universal questions that people ask themselves when they are dying is "Did I matter?" It doesn't matter what your religious beliefs are or if you have no religious beliefs—we all hope that our lives have made a difference. Whether you are interacting with your loved one or are a healthcare professional caring for a patient, this is something that you can help the dying with. Let those who are dying know how they have made a difference in your life. Tell those you care about that you learned something from them, that they made you laugh or that they taught you how to be a better person. People will have a more peaceful death knowing that their lives had a positive effect on this world.

A wonderful ritual you can do with the dying is the rock ceremony. Even if the person is unconscious, you can still do this ritual. Here is how it works. Each person who cares about the dying person gets a small rock, any rock. It can be a special rock they each pick out or just a rock from the garden. One by one, each person walks into the bedroom or hospital room of the patient and lays the rock on the person's chest or lap. As they do this, they should say something like, "This rock represents what you have taught me, done for me, helped me with . . . You have made a difference in my life. Thank you." You will know what to say. Young children can do this ritual as well. They might just say, "I like it when you read to me or take me to the park." It doesn't matter how small or big the statement is—just that the person matters. As each person places the rock on the individual, the person can literally feel the weight of his or her effect on the world. It is a powerful way to say thank you and goodbye. This is just one way to tell people they matter. I am sure you can come up with many ways to show people that you care. And I hope that on the day you die, you will know that you have mattered too. (If you would like a weekly reminder for fun and thoughtful ways to say, "You matter to me," sign up for my "Kindness Reminders," discussed in appendix 4.)

Discrimination at the End of Life for the Mentally Disabled

One significant thing about our healthcare and social service systems that upsets me is that the people we are supposed to be protecting are often not allowed a peaceful, dignified and good death. There can be substantial discrimination at the end of life for those who are mentally disabled. "Wait a minute," you say, "aren't there laws that protect people who are disabled?" Yes, but the laws and regulations can be a double-edged sword and may end up actually harming the patient.

Here is what happens.

A woman has been developmentally disabled for her entire life. She has a family member who is her conservator, and she gets support from a local advocacy group. So the protections are already in place. These protections have worked well during her lifetime, but may cause her problems when it comes time to die. Because she cannot say, "Enough already. I am ready to die," her dying and/or suffering may be prolonged. The doctors hesitate to do what they would do for a "regular" patient, because they don't want to get in trouble. If you or I wanted to stop receiving aggressive treatments, we could just say, "Stop," and the doctors would have to listen to us. But because there are so many legal protections in place, mandating the treatment of the disabled, it is difficult to stop treating this person. And if the patient does not have a strong advocate, then the healthcare professional will feel obligated to prolong the process of dying. This is why having a strong advocate in place may make a difference. There may come a time when you, as the advocate for your loved one, will need to ask for the patient to be allowed the peaceful and pain-free death offered to other patients.

An example of this is seen in the last days of life. As I've described before, when people are near the end, they will probably stop eating because their bodies are no longer able to digest and use food. If you feed a dying person near the very end, the food will likely just sit in the stomach with nowhere to go, and you may be increasing the pain and suffering. For most of us, we will naturally stop eating just before we die. Now, this might be difficult for the people around us to accept, because food often represents love. But eventually our friends and family will make peace with this because they don't want to increase our pain and suffering.

For the mentally disabled patient, however, there are laws that state that these patients must be offered food orally. So we feed the actively dying disabled person even though we would never treat a non-mentally-disabled person that way.

This is what it comes down to: We treat the dying disabled patient different than a non-disabled dying patient. And this can significantly change the dying experience. The laws that protected the individual throughout life may end up causing harm or preventing a peaceful death. At the end of life, we shouldn't treat mentally disabled people as "special" but instead we should treat them as "normal." They are entitled to all of the normal, good care and support we give to other patients during the process of dying. We need to make sure that they receive a referral to hospice, appropriate pain management, grief support, comfort for their suffering and anything else we can do to make the journey more peaceful. This way we can ensure that they get the good death they deserve.

I hope that this end-of-life information will help empower you to make better decisions when the time comes. I would encourage you to seek out more information whenever you have difficult decisions to make. Seeking out information is an important step in the decision making process. Having plenty of information combined with the decision making process you have learned should enable you to be a great decision maker.

Before we finish, we have one more stop on the road together: taking a look at the big picture.

14

The Big Picture

You have come a long way on this journey. You are the person I dedicated this book to: someone who is trying so hard to do right by your loved one. So thank you for being the kind of person who cares. I am privileged that you have allowed me to be a part of your life and the life of your loved one. I hope you will be able to use the tools I have given you and that your decisions start from the heart. As you move forward, I hope that you don't get caught up in all of the questions and the details and forget about the big picture. The big picture is respect and compassion: respect and compassion for your loved one, for the people who care for your loved one, for the healthcare team and especially for yourself. We are all in this together.

Let me share one final story with you.

The Day My Mom Died

Our journey through this book began with my mom, and our journey together will end here, with her story. It has been many years since my mom died, and I have saved the end of her story until now. You have heard the first part of the story, but it is important enough to mention again. After my mom's stroke, she lived for many years in a condition she wouldn't have wanted. It took me a long time to figure out how to do right by my mom. I wasn't able to give her what she needed for many years, but in her final days, I helped give her a good death. I stayed with my mom in the hospital for her last four days. I made sure she had good pain management, got good supportive care and got a chance to say anything else she needed to say. She didn't know that it was me by her side throughout those days and nights, but that was okay. In fact, maybe it made it a little easier.

On the last day of her life, my brother and I got her discharged from the hospital so she could go home with hospice. I was late getting her on hospice. I have learned a lot since then. Looking back, I have to forgive myself for not being able to figure out what was important to her about how she would want to die. I wish I had realized that what was important to her was that she loved her home. Luckily, my brother figured this out and said to me, "She needs to be home to die." So on her last day, the ambulance took her back to her house. My brother and I went ahead and met the ambulance there. Unfortunately, we had many stairs up to the house and the emergency medical technicians needed to wait until another ambulance could arrive so they would have enough men to carry her up the sixteen steps. My brother and I were so worried that she wouldn't make it upstairs in time. We could tell her death was getting closer, as her breathing was changing. Soon the other men arrived and my brother and I got my mom settled in her bed. Even though she was close to death, I could tell she knew she was home. I even said to her, "You are back home." A few minutes later, finally at peace and knowing that her wishes had finally been heard, she died.

I am very grateful that my brother and I had the chance to honor her last wish to be able to die at home. Please make the effort to give voice to your loved one's wishes and to become the best decision maker you can. I have given you the information and tools you need. Now all you have to do is find the courage and strength to do it. I know you can.

Author's Note

Being of Service

I am so grateful to the many wonderful organizations that serve our communities. As a longtime volunteer and supporter of nonprofits, I would encourage you to volunteer and/or financially support the nonprofit organizations in your community that are making a difference in your life. I've listed my favorite nonprofits on the next page, each of which is making a dramatic difference in our world by serving those who are voiceless and need help. You can learn more about these organizations at TheCaregiversPath.com or their respective websites.

Alzheimer's Association

The Alzheimer's Association is the leading voluntary health organization in Alzheimer's care, support and research. It's mission is to eliminate Alzheimer's disease through the advancement of research; to provide and enhance care and support for all those affected; and to reduce the risk of dementia through the promotion of brain health. For more information, visit alz.org.

American Stroke Association

Created in 1997 as a division of the American Heart Association, the American Stroke Association works to improve stroke prevention, diagnosis and treatment to save lives from stroke—America's No. 3 killer and a leading cause of serious disability. To do this, we fund scientific research, help people better understand and avoid stroke, encourage government support, guide healthcare professionals, and provide information to stroke survivors and their caregivers to enhance their quality of life. To learn more, call 1-888-4STROKE or visit strokeassociation.org.

Appendix 1

5 Core Questions Flowchart

1 Does the individual have the ability to make his or her own decisions? Does he or she have decisional capacity?

2b Not Sure

2c Sometimes

2d No

2a Yes

3b Get the person an evaluation to determine capacity

3a Does the person want to make his or her own decisions using autonomy?

4d Yes, the person has capacity

4e Fluctuating

On days when person has capacity, use autonomy; On days when person does not, determine mental age

4f No, the person does not have capacity

4a Yes

4b Yes, along with other loved ones

4c No, even though the person has capacity, he or she would like someone else to be in charge

5 About how old is the person developmentally? What is his or her mental age?

6a 0–6 years old

6b 7–13 years old

6c 14–17 years old

7a Someone else will make all the decisions for the person

7b Use assent to keep the person included in those decisions that are safe to make

7c Do not include the person in the more critical decisions

7d Person can make the less critical decisions

7e Person can make the life-or-death decisions, if person has capacity

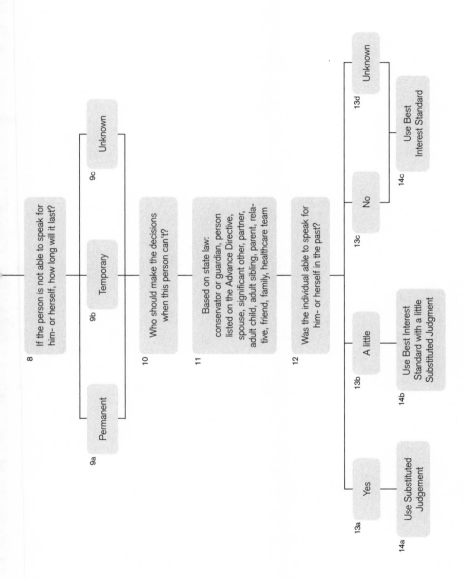

8 If the person is not able to speak for him- or herself, how long will it last?

9a Permanent

9b Temporary

9c Unknown

10 Who should make the decisions when this person can't?

11 Based on state law: conservator or guardian, person listed on the Advance Directive, spouse, significant other, partner, adult child, adult sibling, parent, relative, friend, family, healthcare team

12 Was the individual able to speak for him- or herself in the past?

13a Yes

13b A little

13c No

13d Unknown

14a Use Substituted Judgement

14b Use Best Interest Standard with a little Substituted Judgment

14c Use Best Interest Standard

Appendix 2

An Insider's Guide to Filling Out Your Advance Directive

What is an Advance Directive for Healthcare Decisions? The Advance Directive is a form that a person can complete while she still has the capacity to think and communicate. This form can be used to indicate *who* should make the patient's decisions and *what* the patient would want in different medical situations after the patient loses capacity. Each state has a different form to use, so be sure to get the correct form before you start using this guide. (See Quick Tips for Filling Out Your Advance Directive Form on page 212.)

Most doctors just hand patients the Advance Directive form and tell them to fill it out. But they don't help explain how to use the form or what the decisions mean. I am going to help you think through the process of filling out your Advance Directive.

There are two main decisions you need to make when you are filling out your Advance Directive: *who* you want to make decisions for you and *what* you would want. After I help you with these two questions, I will tell you what to do once you have filled out this form. At the end, I have included instructions on how to find a form that would work in your state.

Whom Should You Pick?

Let's first talk about whom you would want to make decisions for you. In your state, your form might ask you to list your agent, proxy, durable power of attorney for healthcare or surrogate decision maker. (These words all mean the same thing, but different places use different legal terms.) Use the following points to help you make a decision.

1. You should pick someone who is medically literate. What does this mean? The person should be able to understand what the doctor is saying, be able to understand the medical words and be able to understand the medical choices being offered. If the person you thought you were going to pick would be confused by what the doctor would say, then pick someone else.

2. You should pick someone who knows you very well, would know what you would want in a medical crisis and would tell the doctor what you have told her in the past. The person you choose will be asked to listen to medical information and then to use your values to

make medical decisions. The decision maker is not supposed to use her own values, but to speak as if she were you. If the person you thought you would pick wouldn't respect your choices or has very different beliefs from yours, then pick someone else. You want someone who will speak as if she is speaking with your voice, not her own agenda.

3. You should pick someone who won't fall apart in a crisis. It doesn't do you any good if the person is hysterical, can't function or can't stand to visit you in the hospital. You need to pick someone brave enough to be by your side no matter how difficult things get. If the person you thought you would pick doesn't handle his own life very well, then don't have him be in charge of yours.

4. You should pick someone who will do right by you even if it is the most difficult thing she has ever had to do. Sometimes doing the right thing is allowing the person you love to have a peaceful death. Your decision maker needs to be able to live with the difficult decisions she has to make. In reality, she is making the decisions based on what you would want, not what she would want, but that doesn't make it any easier. You have to be able to talk to this person ahead of time about what you would want in different kinds of situations. So if the person you thought you would pick is too afraid to talk about death and dying, then she isn't the right person for this job. Or if she would refuse to follow through with what you have requested, then pick someone else.

5. If you can, pick someone who lives close by or can at least afford to hop on a plane and come to the hospital to

talk to the doctor in person. Too often bad decisions get made because people can't understand that their loved one's condition has changed drastically and that the person is no longer as they remember. If the decision maker can't come right away, perhaps a webcam can be used or a picture can be sent to show what is happening to the patient's body.

6. You can also write down those you *don't* want to be involved in the decision making. The rules regarding who is in charge of you when you are unconscious or incapacitated vary from state to state. You need to protect yourself and choose the person who is right for you.

7. Doctors won't tell you this, but you can pick two or three people to share in your medical decision making. But be careful that you pick people who can work together, who will support each other and who you know won't make things worse for the healthcare team. I had one lady tell me that she picked her two sons to make her decisions and that these two men had never agreed on anything. She is setting herself up for a nightmare, as good decisions won't get made and the doctor will hate having to deal with her sons. You don't want your doctor to hate your decision maker. Please pick carefully.

8. Some people don't pick their spouse, significant other or partner because they know that it would be too much for this person to go through emotionally and that he couldn't make the most difficult decisions. If you do pick your spouse, then you need to be extremely careful about picking alternate decision makers. The alternates will make your decisions if you and your spouse are injured in

the same accident. The alternates should be just as quali-fied as your first choice.

9. The other part of the "who" question is "Whom do you want to be able to receive information about your health?" Because of our HIPAA laws, you now have to state who can and cannot receive your personal informa-tion. Unfortunately, the Advance Directive form doesn't ask this question. I would suggest that you write your choices in the "Other" section of whatever form you are using. Make sure you indicate both those you *do* want to receive your medical information and those you *do not* want to receive your medical information.

Next, let's look at how to tell the doctor what you would want, if you were unable to speak for yourself.

What Would You Want?

1. The first thing to remember is that this form goes into effect when you are unconscious, too mentally disabled or too sedated to speak for yourself. This form will be used when you are injured, sick and/or dying. Too many people, including doctors, think of this form as only a dying form. For some people, this form will be used for years and years because they have become mentally ill or disabled.

2. The next thing to decide is what you would want in certain medical situations. Should you be specific or vague about the specific medical treatments you would want? I would encourage you to be vague. You won't know the exact

medical situation you might find yourself in, and you may guess wrong if you write down "Don't do this" or "Yes, do that." Here is an example: You might have written on your Advance Directive that you would never want to be put on a ventilator. How will this statement be interpreted by the doctors? The doctor will not put you on the ventilator. If he does, it would be considered assault and battery because it is against your will. This recently happened to an elderly gentleman. The gentleman wrote that he didn't want to be hooked up to a ventilator, but what he meant was, he didn't want to live on a ventilator. This became a problem when he needed to be hooked up to a ventilator for four days in order to recover from an infection. He didn't need it forever—just for a few short days. But because he was too specific and had said to never put him on a ventilator, he was not put on life support and he died. So be careful when you request certain medical choices. Make sure that what you have written would work in different situations.

3. So, now that I just scared you, you are probably worried about what to write in this section. I have a solution. It is called a *meaningful recovery statement*. You need to explain to the doctor what kind of life you would want to live if your mind no longer worked well or if it didn't work at all. Now, for some people, any condition is okay, because they believe it is God's will to determine how we live and when we die. But others can't think of anything worse than living in a nursing home, wearing diapers, having other people feed them and not being able to recognize their loved ones. But how will your doctors know what you would want if you don't tell them? Doctors know how to practice medicine. But what they don't

know is what would make for a "meaningful recovery" for you. So you have to tell them.

Here is my meaningful recovery statement:

I value a full life more than a long life. If I have lost the ability to interact with others and have no reasonable chance of regaining this ability, or if my suffering is intense and irreversible, *even though I have no terminal illness*, I do not want to have my life prolonged. I would not then ask to be subjected to surgery or to resuscitation procedures, to intensive care services, or to other life-prolonging measures, including the administration of antibiotics, blood products, or artificial nutrition and hydration. I also believe that the financial and emotional burden on my family should be considered in making these types of decisions.

A few years ago I added this paragraph to my meaningful statement above when I married my husband. That is the great thing about Advance Directives. Over time, you can write a new Advance Directive and modify your wishes as your life and health condition changes.

In general, I do not want to be a burden on my family. I understand that caring for me may not feel like a burden for my husband, at least for a while. So, if he doesn't consider me a burden, whether financial, emotional or other, and he wants me to live for a while in a non-suffering condition while he makes peace with what has happened to me, then that is okay with me. I realize that everyone comes to terms with a loved one's health crisis in their own time and in their own way. I do not want to increase his unhappiness. So if he wants to care for me for a period of time, because that is less painful than letting me go, then that is okay with me. He is allowed to say, "Enough," when he is ready.

Because I have written this in my Advance Directive, the doctors will know what is important to me. Of course, this doesn't have to be your statement. Write one that is meaningful to you and attach it to or write it on your Advance Directive.

One more thing: Please address the issue of terminal versus non-terminal situations. If you are terminal, then it is important your doctors know where and how you would want to die. If you are severely disabled but are not going to die soon, then you need to let them know what kind of life would be tolerable for you. The best way to be protected is to write it down.

We have gone over the main sections of the Advance Directive. Of course, you can write down anything else you want the doctors to know about you. You might want to tell them if you would like to donate your organs or if you are for or against an autopsy. This is your form, so write down whatever works for you.

I encourage families to have Advance Directive gatherings where everyone gets together to talk about what they would want while filling out their Advance Directives together. This is a great way to make sure that as a group, your family and friends have heard and understood your wishes.

Now That You Have Filled It Out, What Should You Do Next?

1. Well, the first thing you have to do is sit down with your primary and your alternate decision makers and discuss what you would want if you were injured, disabled or dying. Remember that this form goes into effect when you are unconscious, too mentally disabled or too sedated to speak for yourself.

2. Then, you need to give all of your decision makers a copy of your Advance Directive. You also need to give copies to all your doctors and your local hospital. You should keep a copy at home either by your bedside, taped to the inside of your medicine cabinet or on your refrigerator so the paramedics can find it. You can also keep one in your car or in your purse. You might want to take the form on vacation with you. People won't know what you want if they can't find your instructions. Doctors get frustrated when the family says, "The patient has an Advance Directive, but we don't know where it is." What I do is keep a paper in my wallet saying where to find my Advance Directive and whom to call in case of an emergency. (Please *don't* keep your only copy in your safe deposit box, where only you can get it.)

3. The next time you go to your doctor, bring him a copy and discuss what you have written. Ask your doctor if he would be willing to respect your choices. This is where you can really get into trouble. Some doctors won't follow what people have written in their Advance Directive, so you better know right now if yours is one of those doctors. Also, some doctors are too afraid to talk about death. If you don't think your doctor will respect your wishes or if he is too uncomfortable talking about dying, then find yourself another doctor. I am serious about this. Doctors go against people's instructions and prolong the suffering and dying of patients in every hospital. If you find yourself in this situation, with the doctor refusing to follow your Advance Directive, then the bioethics committee at the hospital should be able to help you. If you

have been chosen as the decision maker and are unwilling to follow what is written in the Advance Directive, then you shouldn't be the decision maker. Remove yourself and have the doctors use one of the alternates.

How to Get an Advance Directive

1. The easiest way to get a free Advance Directive is to go to the front desk of any hospital. Just tell them you need one or more for your family, and they should give the forms to you for free.

2. You can go online to caringinfo.org for a free, state-specific form. These forms are also available on many other organizations' websites. Just type in the words "Advance Directive" and the name of the state where you live, and plenty of options should appear.

3. You can also order an Advance Directive form called Five Wishes from agingwithdignity.org. This is a very good document for explaining what you would want in certain situations. There are forms in twenty-three different languages, including Braille, and they are valid in forty states. The document costs $5 and can be ordered in bulk (twenty-five copies or more are $1 each) at 888-5-WISHES or agingwithdignity.org.

4. Your doctor's office should have Advance Directive forms available, but unfortunately, many doctors don't keep them in their offices.

Do You Want to Make Your Own Decisions Even When You Have Capacity?

Now that your Advance Directive is complete, you may want to tell your doctor whether or not you want to make your own medical decisions starting right now, while you still have capacity. For some people and in some cultures, the patient would like to have someone else make the decisions even though the individual has full capacity and the ability to make his or her own decisions. If this is important to you, you will want to answer the question below and then use one of the three options on the following pages to document your wishes. Copy the option page that is right for you; then fill it out and give it to your doctor.

Do you want to make your own medical decisions?

- Yes, I want to be in charge of receiving my medical information and making my own decisions.

- Yes, but I don't want to make the decision alone:

  - I will make the decision together with other people. (Use Option 1 on page 208 to clarify your wishes.)

  - I will make the final decision, but I will want advice from other people. (Use Option 2 on page 209 to clarify your wishes.)

- No, I don't want to make my own medical decisions. I want someone else to handle the decision making starting now, even though I have the ability to decide for myself. (Use Option 3 on page 210 to clarify your wishes.)

Option 1

Yes, I want to make my own medical decisions, with the help of the following people (write in the names of those you will consult):

My spouse _____

My significant other _____

My partner _____

My family _____

_____

My doctor(s) _____

_____

My religious leader(s) _____

My community leader(s) _____

My friends _____

_____

Others _____

_____

The following people should *not* be involved in my medical decision making:

_____

_____

_____

Signature _____

Date _____

Option 2

I will make all final medical decisions, but I will want advice from other people, including (write in the names of those you will consult):

My spouse _____

My significant other _____

My partner _____

My family _____

_____

My doctor(s) _____

_____

My religious leader(s) _____

My community leader(s) _____

My friends _____

_____

Others _____

_____

The following people should *not* be involved in my medical decision making:

_____

_____

_____

Signature _____

Date _____

Option 3

No, I do not want to make my own medical decisions. I want someone else to handle the decision making for me, even though I have the ability to decide for myself (decisional capacity). I realize I can get back the power to make my own decisions just by telling my doctor, as long as I still have decisional capacity at that time. I want the following person/people to make my decisions for me starting now:

My spouse _____

My significant other _____

My partner _____

My family _____

_____

My doctor(s) _____

_____

My religious leader(s) _____

My community leader(s) _____

My friends _____

_____

Others _____

_____

The following people should *not* be involved in my medical decision making:

_____

_____

_____

Signature _____

Date _____

[Note: This next section is optional. I am including it here for the sake of your doctors. Some healthcare professionals are not used to people not wanting to make their own decisions while they can think for themselves. Personally, I have met lots of people who have asked someone else to make their decisions for them, even while they could still speak for themselves. This information will help the doctor respect your wishes. (Even though the doctor should respect your wishes without you explaining, we might as well make it easier for him or her.)]

Here are some of the reasons I would like someone else to make my decisions (circle all the answers that apply):

I don't want to worry about making the decisions.

I want to focus on getting better.

This is the way we do things in my culture.

This is the way we do things in my family.

This is the way we do things in my religion.

I don't have the energy to do all the necessary research to make a good decision.

I don't think I would be a good decision maker.

I just don't want to make the decisions.

I don't want to tell you why.

Other _____

_____

Signature _____

Date _____

Quick Tips for Filling Out Your Advance Directive Form

Whom should you pick?
1. Pick someone who will understand what the doctor is saying.
2. Pick someone who knows you well and has listened to what you want.
3. Pick someone who won't fall apart in a crisis.
4. Pick someone who will do what you have asked, even if it difficult to do.
5. Pick someone who is close by geographically.
6. Write down whom you don't want to be involved in the decision making.
7. You can pick two or three people to work together as your decision makers.
8. Your spouse, significant other or partner may not be your best choice, and you may want to choose someone else.
9. In the "Other" section of the form, state whom you do and don't want to be told your medical information.

What would you want?
1. This form goes into effect when your brain isn't working anymore, not just when you are dying.
2. Don't be too specific about the particular treatments you want or don't want, because you don't know what the medical situation will be when you need this form.
3. Write out a meaningful recovery statement describing what kind of life you would want if you were disabled and couldn't think anymore.
4. Tell the doctors what they should do if you were going to live in a terrible condition, as well as what you would want if you were dying.
5. Write down anything else you want your doctors and loved ones to know about where or how you want to die, organ donation preferences or autopsy instructions.

Make sure that your decision makers, your doctors and the hospital get copies of your form and that you talk about it with those who will be involved in your care.

Appendix 3

Action Questions

Action Questions

1. What is the approximate mental age of the individual *today*?
2. Is this person able to make his or her own decisions?
3. If the person can't make his or her own decisions, will this lack of decision making ability continue or is it only temporary?
4. If the lack of capacity will only be for a short period of time, does this decision need to be made today or can I wait to see if he or she will regain the ability soon?
5. How important and serious is this decision?
6. Who should make the decisions while he or she has lost capacity?
7. Should this individual be involved in making this decision? If so, how much?
8. Was the person able to think and communicate in the past, and if so, was he or she fully capable or just partially capable?
9. Am I going to use Substituted Judgment or the Best Interest Standard?
10. What are the person's quality-of-life goals and what would he or she say in this situation?
11. How can I keep the person included in ways that are safe for him or her to participate?
12. What other questions should I use from the checklists in this book?

Appendix 4

"Kindness Reminders"

The "Kindness Reminder" is a brief weekly email to remind you to connect with your aging parent or other loved ones. Each reminder is full of touching and fun ways to reach out and connect.

When a colleague asked me to create these reminders for him, I realized I have been doing this type of thing all my life. I used to call some of my brothers and remind them to call our dad. It wasn't that they didn't care; it was just that like all of us, we get caught up in our own lives.

People think I am amazing because I remember to call on birthdays or to call once a week to check on my elders. I am not amazing; I am organized. I book recurring appointments in my PDA so that it sends me reminders to call, write or somehow show I care. Otherwise, it would slip my mind and weeks would go by before I would make the effort.

These reminders will give you a number of ways to show your concern and your love. I will also give you ideas for how to thank those who are taking care of your loved one when you are either far away or otherwise unable to be there. The more you show appreciation for those who take care of your loved one, the better care he or she will get. Here is an example:

Week 30: Take the person back to the old neighborhood
One of the best trips my dad ever had was when my brother took him back to visit his old neighborhood. Not only was this a gift for my dad but for my brother as well. The pictures from this trip are full of joy. My dad was so happy to be able to share this with his son.

If your loved one is able, take them on a trip—even if it's only for the day. Take the person while he or she is still able to travel. Your loved one only has so many healthy days left; spend them wisely. If he or she can't get out, use Google Earth to show your loved one how the town looks today.

Sign up for this free service at KindEthics.com or TheCaregiversPath.com. Thanks for helping me make the world a **kind**er place.

Glossary

Advance Directive: A written document that indicates what types of medical treatment you would want and whom the doctor should talk to when you are unable to speak for yourself. This document is a combination of a Living Will and a Durable Power of Attorney for Healthcare.

Agent: The person the doctor should talk to regarding healthcare decisions when the patient is unable to speak for him-or herself. Other terms include *durable power of attorney for healthcare, proxy* and *surrogate decision maker*.

AND: Stands for *allow natural death*, which is another way to say *do not resuscitate*. An AND is a request to *not* have cardio-pulmonary resuscitation (CPR) if your heart stops and/or if you stop breathing.

Assent: Asking an individual who has limited capacity, similar to someone with a developmental age of seven to thirteen years, if he or she would agree to participate in a test, treatment or surgery. Assent means the person agrees to participate (see *Dissent* for information about when the person does not agree).

Autonomy: When a person with decisional capacity is allowed to make the decisions about what will happen to his or her own body.

Best Interest Standard: The standard that applies when the patient has lost capacity and we don't know what this person would want and/or the patient doesn't have any loved ones to say what the patient would want. In this case, we make decisions as best we can.

Capacity: When the patient has the mental ability to make his or her own decisions.

Consent: See *informed consent*.

Competent or **competency**: A legal term to describe when a person has the ability to make his or her own decisions.

Conservator: A court-appointed person who is assigned to make decisions for an incapacitated person. This person may also be called a *guardian*. The conservator may be in charge of medical decisions, financial decisions or both.

CPR: Stands for *cardiopulmonary resuscitation*, which is attempted if your heart stops and/or if you stop breathing.

Decision Making Framework: The Decision Making Framework has three parts: Autonomy, Substituted Judgment and the Best Interest Standard. You will need to choose the correct framework for the person you are caring for in order to be respectful of the individual's wishes. This is the starting point for all good decision making.

Decisional capacity: When the patient has the mental ability to make his or her own decisions.

Dissent: When we ask the individual who has limited capacity, similar to someone with a developmental age of seven to thirteen years, if he or she would agree to participate in a test, treatment or surgery, and the person says no or does not agree to participate (see *Assent* for information about when the person agrees).

DNAR: Stands for do not *attempt* resuscitation. A DNAR is a request to *not* have cardiopulmonary resuscitation (CPR) if your heart stops and/or if you stop breathing.

DNR: Stands for *do not resuscitate*. A DNR is a request to *not* have cardiopulmonary resuscitation (CPR) if your heart stops and/or if you stop breathing.

Durable Power of Attorney for Finances: This term is used to describe both the document that says who should be in charge of your financial decisions when you are unable to make your own decisions and the person who is making these decisions. This document does not include information about who will have medical decision making power.

Durable Power of Attorney for Healthcare: This term is used to describe both the document that says who should be in charge of your healthcare decisions when you are unable to make your own decisions and the person who is making these decisions. Other terms include *agent, proxy* and s*urrogate decision maker*. This document does not include information about who will have financial decision making power.

Fluctuating capacity: When the patient sometimes has the mental ability to make his or her own decisions and sometimes does not have the ability.

Guardian: A court-appointed person who is assigned to make decisions for an incapacitated person. This person may also be called a *conservator*. The guardian may be in charge of medical decisions, financial decisions or both.

HIPAA: Stand for Health Information Portability and Accountability Act. This law protects your medical information. It also allows you to say who will and will not have access to your personal health information.

Informed consent or informed refusal: A doctor has to give a patient or a decision maker enough information so that a good, informed decision can be made regarding the treatment options. The decision maker can either consent to or refuse the recommended treatment options.

Living Will: A written document that indicates what types of medical treatment are desired. A Living Will can be very specific or very general. This document may also be called an *Advance Directive*.

POLST: Stands for Physician Orders for Life-Sustaining Treatments, which is a doctor's order form that documents the patient's wishes, not only about CPR but for other end-of-life choices. When you have a POLST form, your wishes will be respected whether you are in the hospital, the ambulance, a long-term care facility or your home. In your area, this form may have a slightly different name, such as MOLST, or Medical Orders for Life-Sustaining Treatments. The POLST form may or may not be available where you live.

Power of attorney for healthcare: See *Durable Power of Attorney for Healthcare*.

Proxy: The person the doctor should talk to regarding healthcare decisions when the patient is unable to speak for him or herself. Other terms include *agent, durable power of attorney for healthcare* and *surrogate decision maker*.

Shared Decision Making Model: The Shared Decision Making Model will tell us whether or not a person should be a participant in the decision making process and how big of a voice he or she should have in making the decisions.

Sliding Scale for Decision Making: The Sliding Scale for Decision Making tells us that the more serious the risks involved in the decision, the more the person needs the ability to think and communicate in order to be involved in the decision making process. A less risky decision requires less capacity on the part of the patient, while a more risky decision requires more capacity if the patient is to be involved.

Substituted Judgment: When someone else makes the medical decisions for a person who has lost capacity, based on the values and wishes of the patient.

Surrogate decision maker: The person the doctor should talk to regarding healthcare decisions when the patient is unable to speak for him or herself. Other terms include *agent, durable power of attorney for healthcare* and *proxy.*

Unbefriended: A term used to describe someone who doesn't have any friends or loved ones whom the doctor can talk to about the patient and the patient's values when the patient has lost capacity. Same as *Unrepresented.*

Unrepresented: A term used to describe someone who doesn't have any friends or loved ones whom the doctor can talk to about the patient and the patient's values when the patient has lost capacity. Same as *Unbefriended.*

Acknowledgments

Thank you to Greenleaf: Tanya Hall, thanks for finding me on LinkedIn and bringing me to Greenleaf; my editors, Bill Crawford and Lari Bishop; my production manager, Chris McRay; my cover designer, Lisa Woods; my proofreader, Amy McIlwaine; my compositor, Kim Scott; my technical artist, Brian Phillips; and Sheila Parr, my art director. You rock!

I want to thank all the people who care for our loved ones. I am so grateful to the people who work in our hospitals, doctor's offices, long-term care facilities and group homes. Thanks also to the home health nurses, the hospice nurses and the private caregivers in our homes. Thanks for doing all that you do.

Thanks to those who have taught me so much academically, professionally and personally. Thank you for teaching me what I needed to know to arrive at this point in my life.

I want to give a special thank-you to all the people who have told me their stories and allowed me to help them along their way. It is a gift to be able to be of service to you.

My heart is full of gratitude to the families that have allowed me in to help their loved ones die. It has been an honor and a privilege to be present with you and your loved ones during their last days.

I especially want to thank those who helped read the early drafts of this book and gave me great advice: Bonnie Thomas,

Carol Breslin, Dr. Phil Oncley, Kathy Terry, Anita Miller, Aurora Morales, Maria Bratly and Dale Carter.

Thank you to my loved ones who gave me the opportunity to be a caregiver and to learn new ways to love. It was exhausting and fulfilling.

A special thank-you to my brothers for supporting me through the difficult days we shared on our journey together. It wasn't easy for any of us to be so young and to have to deal with so much. Thanks for being there.

Thanks to my mom for teaching me the difficult lessons.

Thanks to my dad for making it easy.

And finally, I want to thank Ed You, my husband, my best friend, and my biggest cheerleader. I wouldn't have been able to write this without your love and support. Thanks for reading all the different drafts along the way. You are my super-hero.

References

Connor, S.R., B. Pyenson, K. Fitch, C. Spence, and K. Iwasaki. 2007. Comparing hospice and nonhospice patient survival among patients who die within a three-year window. *Journal of Pain and Symptom Management* 33 (3).

Diem, S. J., J. D. Lantos, and J. A. Tulsky. 1996. Cardiopulmonary resuscitation on television: Miracles and misinformation. *New England Journal of Medicine* 334 (24): 1578–82.

Ehlenbach, W.J., A.E. Barnato, J.R. Curtis, et al. 2009. Epidemiologic study of hospital cardiopulmonary resuscitation in the elderly. *New England Journal of Medicine* 361 (1): 22–31.

Gordon, S. 2009. CPR Survival Rates for Older People Unchanged. *HealthDay: News for Healthier Living*, July 1, 2009.

Kaldjian, L.C., Z.D. Erekson, T.H. Haberle, et al. 2009. Code status discussion and goals of care among hospitalized adults. *Journal of Medical Ethics* 35 (6): 338–42.

Peberdy, M.A., W. Kaye, J.P. Ornato, et al. 2003. Cardiopulmonary resuscitation of adults in the hospital: A report of 14,720 cardiac arrests from the National Registry of Cardiopulmonary Resuscitation. *Resuscitation* 58 (3): 297–308.

Index

About the Author

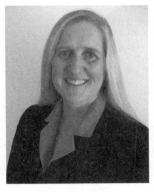 Viki Kind, MA, is a clinical bioethicist, medical educator, and hospice volunteer. She is a renowned lecturer, who inspires healthcare professionals throughout the United States to have integrity and compassion and teaches them techniques to improve communication about end-of-life care. She is the co-creator of the nationally distributed DVD, *The Trusted Advisor: Relate, Respect and Respond*, which focuses on improving the senior patient's medical experience. Patients, families, and healthcare professionals have come to rely on Viki's practical approach to dealing with challenging healthcare dilemmas.

Viki provides bioethics consultation and support for many hospitals in the Los Angeles area. She is also a member of the Los Angeles County Bar Association's Bioethics Committee and the Southern California Bioethics Committee Consortium. She holds a master's degree in bioethics from the Medical College of Wisconsin and a bachelor's degree in speech communication from California State University at Northridge. She also has specialized training in mediation and cultural negotiation from Pepperdine University and UCLA.

Viki resides in Los Angeles with her husband, Ed, and her cat, BooBoo.

For more information about Viki, *The Caregiver's Path to Compassionate Decision Making: Making Choices for Those Who Can't*, and the topics of bioethics, visit www.kindethics.com and www.thecaregiverspath.com.